NERVOUS AND MENTAL DISEASE MONOGRAPHS. No. 65

Sketches in Psychosomatic Medicine

BY

SMITH ELY JELLIFFE, M.D.

CONSULTING NEUROLOGIST TO MANHATTAN STATE AND
KINGS PARK HOSPITALS, NEW YORK

British Library Cataloguing-in-Publication Data
A catalogue record for this book is available from the
British Library

Dedicated to A. A. Brill, M.D., to whom I am mostly indebted for my introduction to the Freudian conceptions.

CONTENTS

INTRODUCTION

I have brought together these few papers under the caption of
"Sketches in Psychosomatic Medicine" to gratify my own satisfaction in having written them, and to further the conviction that they
have been worth while and the hope that they will be of service in
the understanding and therapy of similar and related conditions still
imperfectly dealt with in medical practice.

The general ideas stem from the Socratic principle of the wholeness
of the body and as related in Plato's Charmides, " one looks to the
cure of the ' soul ' in order to cure the body."

Freud for the first time rendered the " soul " accessible to conscious
perception and offered a method for gaining insight into dynamic
principles of creative and destructive tendencies without which no
real psychosomatic unity is understandable.

Whereas the principles involved are derivations from others, a
modest claim for originality in the application of these conceptions
to the study of specific medical situations is made. I do not need to
accent this further than Freud's own bracketing of these efforts and
those of Groddeck as novel and important.

From an actual historical point of view my earlier papers were
written before I knew of Groddeck's work, in which latter the principles here worked out at times in considerable detail are but suggested in Groddeck's intriguing contributions.

It is furthermore of considerable satisfaction to present this group
of studies. When I brought some of these and related papers before
my neuropsychiatric confréres, psychoanalytic and otherwise, at the
best they were received in conservative silence. Today psychosomatic medicine is almost a byword of progress. Thus I lay my
offering before the Temple of Aesculapius with the fond hope it may
find favor in the eyes of my colleagues. Should this prove to be so,
as these are but a portion of related studies, I may find courage to
collect others in the form these have achieved.

I.

WHAT PRICE HEALING?

A FRAGMENTARY INQUIRY *

A recent striking experience has convinced me that its outlining may not be amiss. It deals with a situation that has been repeated several times in my clinical work. I would also briefly report two other cases of related significance and thus offer a contribution to the conception or idea that not infrequently an acute or even a chronic psychosis may follow the " cure," surgical chiefly, of a longstanding irreversible somatic disorder. There are a number of valuable theoretical considerations underlying this general situation, enough in my opinion to justify the fragmentary presentation of these three cases.

Case 1.—A colleague asked me to consult with him about " Miss G." She was suffering from a mild agitated depression. She had made one attempt at suicide by illuminating gas and had hovered dangerously near to a window ten stories above the ground. She had been acting queerly only about two or three weeks.

I obtained the following history, abbreviated so as to present the salient features:

Her father was Irish, her mother American. They were of the pioneer type, having settled in the Rockies where, in one of the leading western cities, the father built up a large and profitable business, one of the first in those days following the forty-niners. The oldest daughter, now sixty-six, was born there. A second daughter, the patient, now sixty-four, was born in the East; also a son, who would have been sixty-two.

The father, having made his " pile," moved East, settled down, and the three children were brought up decorously in one of our " quietest " of cities. The oldest girl was the lively one and is even now an active, loquacious, Irish type, still comely. The second girl was always a bit retiring. She was sweet and dutiful but was " nervous." She played the piano nicely and sang. She must have been quite pretty, as she is still a good looking woman. The son was a healthy boy. He married, had no children, and died at fifty-three of an apoplectic stroke. The older sister was married at twenty-three but at thirty was left a widow. Having no children she returned to the family home.

At eighteen the patient made a runaway match against her parents'

* Reprinted by permission from the *Journal of the American Medical Association*, May 3, 1930, Vol. 94, pp. 1393–1395.

wishes. Apparently it was a great disappointment to her, as she returned home in less than a year, gave birth to a dead child, divorced her husband two years later, and remained at home. In 1912 the father and mother died at advanced ages, seventy-nine and seventy-six, and the two sisters lived on in the old home, much attached to each other, the younger being dependent on her more dominant, breezy, active widowed sister. About six years ago they moved to New York. Their father's estate, in trust, left them modest but comfortable incomes. They did their own house-keeping, the patient usually doing the cooking, and they lived simply but nicely in a well appointed apartment on the West Side. They were much alone and apparently no men bothered them.

The family history reveals little. The father had diabetes and both the father and mother were of a nervous disposition.

As stated, the patient was a quiet, pleasing child. She was born normally, developed well, walked and talked at the proper time, and was able to read at five. She had measles and mumps. She was bright, and showed no neurotic traits in childhood. She attended public and private schools until she was eighteen, when she made the marriage which apparently did not work. There were no other illnesses of any nature. She was 5 feet 3 inches (160 cm.) in height and of late years had grown heavy, weighing 180 pounds (81.6 Kg.).

She had one difficulty, however, which constitutes the main point of this story. I was unable to determine from her just when it began, but the sister thought she had had it from childhood. She had to urinate at least every fifteen or twenty minutes. Since her marriage and the birth of the child it had been a chronic complaint, and in spite of all methods of treatment, not pursued with any great regularity, it had persisted. Naturally, her life was greatly hampered. She rarely went out, and if she did, only along certain specified routes where she knew she could find relief. In the earlier years the urinary urge had not been quite so frequent. This disorder tied her all the more to the sister, and they had lived their quiet lives alone for the past sixteen years.

Four months previous to my seeing her, my colleague was told about the bladder trouble, the patient had always been reticent, and he recognized its neurotic nature. He did not, however, endeavor to study its functional meaning or its value, and proposed gradual bladder dilation as a cure. The bladder was certainly very much contracted, as the roentgen examination demonstrated. He began with gradual dilation by fluids, and after six or seven weeks, was able to double the size of the bladder, so that the patient could retain the urine for about four or five hours.

Shortly thereafter there began to be a gradual increase in restlessness and sleeplessness. The patient began to have a tense, worried look. Still she made no complaints. Then her sister noted more and more a hunted look on her face and the gradually increasing sign of worry and anxiety. At first no definite worries came to consciousness.

Then one day the sister found the patient in the kitchen sitting before the oven of the gas stove with the gas escaping, her head partly thrust into the oven. The patient complained of being worried. The anxious, harried look increased, and a week or so later the patient began to edge up close to an open window and was leaning out when the sister pulled her back. All this time she was very quiet and but two series of ideas kept coming in her mind:

1. *She had a plate of some false teeth in the upper jaw. She was constantly worrying lest she lose a tooth that partly held the plate, so that the plate would drop out. This preoccupied her mind.*

2. *Also she worried lest her sister and she would get into trouble at the bank. She kept the accounts of their joint housekeeping, jotting down all their expenditures on a piece of paper from day to day. The sister drew the monthly checks to pay them. Her anxiety would center about the fact that she feared she had omitted some of the items. This would get them in trouble at the bank—what trouble she could not state. It was just a vague anxiety.*

On examination there were no outstanding neurologic anomalies. The pupillary reflexes were prompt and ample; the eyeballs moved freely, and there were no paralyses, speech disturbances or reflx disturbancs anywhere. The blood pressure was average. There were no toxic signs.

The patient was quiet, plainly anxious, and regarded me somewhat askance but answered questions and told me of her ideas in a low voice slightly slowed. All her movements were slowed, but she said that ideas raced through her head. She had no uncomfortable bodily sensations and apparently no hallucinations. She did not care to eat, but did eat and slept fitfully.

She presented the typical appearance of an involutional depression with anxiety.

From a whole group of possibilities in the interpretation of this case I wish to pick on one set of factors which constitutes the point to be emphasized in this presentation. As the other cases to be reported briefly show related situations, I believe I am justified in narrowing the search for the meaning of the psychosis to the factor to be mentioned.

When her physician cured this patient of her bladder trouble, quite unwittingly he took away something of vital importance to her. In a manner of speaking, he deprived her of her functional baby. In more strictly psychoanalytic terms he displaced, routed out, a source of unconscious erotic gratification. Where did it go? Briefly, into the psychosis!

This cannot be understood completely at this time. It is not necessary. One has but to recall that the " anxiety " is to be regarded as a defense chiefly against the emergence into consciousness of a forbidden type of erotic gratification. When the patient had her enuresis at hand to provide the gratification, even if its erotic quality was not appreciated, she was able to function, in view of the limited calls on her personality. Her little round of household duties did not demand much, and her instinctual needs on the libidinous side had since childhood found a primitive source of fixation. It was evident that the hasty marriage was a futile gesture, the dead child served as a throw back, and the enuresis had played the rôle of a complete sexual equivalent. It probably fulfilled the full scale from urethral to masturbatory and coitus needs. No effort is here made to attempt to prove all these contentions. Only one point may be offered in partial substantiation so far as the masturbatory substitution is concerned.

As is well recognized in modern and even in ancient psychopathology as so known, delusional or even an obsessional mental state may be conceived of as having the same construction as a dream. Hence the fear of a tooth falling out can be put into the dream form. For years analyses have shown that dreams of tooth pulling and of teeth falling out have had masturbatory significance. Hence in applying this empiric finding to the patient's fear, one may say that, with the deprivation of the enuretic gratification, one of the things it covered up and gratified was a masturbatory wish. Now this craving threatened to come into consciousness and the censorship repressed it by anxiety. It is not necessary here to go into the whole argument about the validity of this conception and all the reasons attached to it.[1]

It has been proved over and over again, especially when a symptom in an hysterical person was supposed to have been cured, as a paralysis was by electricity, for instance, that it simply found a resting place, a displacement in some other part of the body. Numerous types of such displacements are known, and, unfortunately, even in so-called psychoanalysis, chiefly by lay-analysts who are ignorant of the " body " and the psychic body scheme (Schilder), a conversion symptom, of often less significant nature, may be dispelled, with the result that the unanalyzed part of the individual's illness appears in another type of manifestation. A conversion symptom may prove the most economical and least dangerous type of symptom for a psychoneurosis to assume. But it is not my purpose to enter this complicated field further than to state that psychotherapy of disturbances of chiefly psychogenic origin is a most vital and important kind of therapy. " Fools rush in where angels fear to tread " is more true of psychotherapy than of any other form of therapy.

[1] Freud: Inhibition, Anxiety, and Symptom (English translation). W. W. Norton & Co.

It is interesting to note that, when medicine began to come out of the medieval quagmire, the first important restrictions were placed on surgical activities. Next the giving of medicines was accounted practice of medicine. At the present status of the actual laws of most of our states, anyone can practice psychotherapy; that is, interfere with the most complex and most important of all human activities. During the late war a man with flat feet was excused from being even a private, but a man with a flat head might even be made a colonel. Such are the inconsistencies of life. " What fools we mortals be! "

Case 2.—Several years ago there came into my office an alert, neatly dressed, evidently well set up man of about forty. He was married, I gathered, but he was so reticent, first giving an assumed name, a false address and falsifying certain facts, that I was intrigued.

He was quite desirous that I should not make any notes of his case and only consented to my carrying out my usual routine when I showed him that I wrote my histories in a cryptic manner. I had certain arbitrary personal signs for certain things. I often introduced foreign words into the history. I used the Morse code and several languages and, showing him some lines of what he had told me, asked him to translate. Thus a confidence, not his, may I remark, might look like this:

which meant that the " patient went to a certain house the day before, met a man, had intercourse three times by rectum, and two weeks later had a chancre." Still he was not fully relieved, so I desisted and listened and wrote my history from memory later in the evening.

It did not take long to see that this was a case of a subtle beginning paranoia, with delusional ideas of jealousy, suspiciousness, and some miserliness in a very neat person, with evident indication of the anal-erotic character in a fine type of individual.

The whole process had begun within three weeks after he had had a successful dilation of a functional esophageal stricture (cardiospasm).

I was unable to follow this case and cannot give a detailed history according to my notes, for he asked for the history notes as they contained, he said, some interesting literary material that he wished to work up, and " Mr. Green " departed from my professional horizon. When I see him at rare intervals in the Plaza grill, he dodges behind conveniently situated waiters.

I could write a book about the third case, as I have known the patient since our mutual childhoods. It was not the first I had observed but it was most striking. I shall present only a brief history.

Case 3.—The father had been in the wholesale liquor business and was prosperous. The mother, beautiful and socially aspiring, had persuaded him to give up business; he retired in comfortable circumstances and soon died. There were four children. The oldest son, when about twenty-four, a handsome, charming dilettante, fell in love with an attractive divorcée. Church circles regarded her with suspicion. There was some trouble and he committed suicide. My patient, the next child, was a bright and lively girl, active in church circles, and much admired for her verve, beauty and financial prospects. Her younger brother was a chum of a younger brother close to me. The youngest girl, a beautiful child of twelve or thirteen, died suddenly from what was rumored to be an imperforate hymen with septic poisoning. This was the setting when I was sixteen and first knew the family. They were all close friends of my mother. It was a sad household by reason of the suicide of the oldest brother and the sudden death of the young girl.

Then there were vague rumors that the remaining daughter, now eighteen or twenty, was having difficulty in eating, and during the years I was studying medicine I learned that she regurgitated her food and became thin and gaunt, and was a cause of much anxiety at home. This continued, and I heard of her from time to time. At about twenty-five or twenty-six she married an older man, a dealer in second hand building material, well to do but close, and they had one son. The brother I now saw infrequently and heard rumors of periodic depressions alternating or interspersed with digestive disturbances.

Thus one may easily realize that there was something neurotic about the whole family. In this connection its further outlining on hereditary patterns is, I believe, unimportant.

Later I learned, after I was definitely asked to consult in the case, what I had already heard rumors of, that the girl had developed an esophageal diverticulum into which her food would first settle. When she had filled this she could eat and get food in the stomach. Later the fermentation in the diverticulum would cause regurgitation, and so she went on for years, a chronic, thin, unhappy invalid, making her social rounds and attempting to carry on, for she had a lot of determination.

All this time innumerable attempts were made to effect a cure, but all were unsuccessful and she avoided a radical operation. Then, as far as I can reconstruct the history, two events occurred, more or less in close time relationship. The patient went to the X Clinic and was " cured," and the United States went into the war and her son volunteered.

She developed at first an acute anxiety situation with periods of wild restlessness. I saw her in the early stages, soon after her return from her healing process and before the most significant phases of her psychosis had broken through. It was then I was able to get some dream material and see what the esophageal diverticulum had stood for. I cannot go into this material now in detail; I must be granted my own interpretation. Needless to say, the father fixation was loaded, had passed to the suicidal brother, and had inaugurated the original regurgitation; rejection by neurotic conversion. The younger brother, handsome like his dead brother, entered into the picture as well. The marriage had held and had provided the opportunity for some psychosexual evolution, but the unsublimated part of the father cathexis now grew more and more diverted to the growing son. Among the dream fragments, the son figured distinctly on the Jocasta model.

Then when the son actually went to Europe, albeit in a distinctly diplomatic and noncombatant rôle, the psychosis took on a violent form. The patient attempted suicide by cutting her wrists. One dramatic escape out of a window which brought in the entire fire department of the district antedated her going to an institution, where after two or three years in strict confinement she made a social recovery and since then had improved, especially with the death of her husband, always an ambivalent factor in her anal eroticism. With the marriage of the son with two children at present, she has come more or less into placid waters.

Now the nub of this communication, to which I could add others in other gastrointestinal fields stripped of many ifs and buts and ands, is to show what has been suggested by many another before me: that a chronic neurotic disorder is capable of building up definite tissue alterations in various organs of the body to satisfy through libidinal cathexis a *status quo* between the respective claims of the Id, the Ego and the Super-Ego. The primary organ neurosis, at first reversible and susceptible of cure or amelioration before the age of forty, by this time approximately had become irreversible, and what is designated as an organic disease. No amount of psychoanalysis can change the situation now and usually surgical therapy is needed.

When the patient by such therapy is cured of the organic disorder, *without concomitant psychotherapy,* and assuming that it has been a progressive cathectic process, then a pathologic displacement, substitution, projection or other type of mechanism is imperative. When the organism as a whole is not in adjustment and the brake, or eddy, or inhibiting investment has been released, a frozen credit becomes a liquid asset, as in the present instances, and the pressure is too great for the Ego. Like the greedy investors who attempted to invest their paper liquid profits on a margin, in the recent stock debacle, down goes the whole defense and the psychotic adjustment becomes imperative.

II.

PSYCHOPATHOLOGY AND ORGANIC DISEASE *

Just at this point in this symposium might I introduce the story of two rather well inebriated citizens who would witness a wrestling match at the Madison Square Garden in New York City. As they entered and took their seats, Londos and his opponent were in a clinch. After about 10–15 minutes one of these visitors looking up and noting Londos still in a clinch, said, " Come on, Joe, let's go out, here's where we came in."

I am not certain that my tale is quite *a propos* save as to that aspect of my reappearance on the platform wherein it might seem that " here's where you came in "—and maybe your state of bewilderment may more properly follow my remarks rather than have preceded them.

You have listened to two important aspects of psychopathology and psychotherapy—Prophylaxis in Childhood and Adolescence, by Dr. Williams, and the Psychoneuroses and Psychoses, by Dr. Brill. I would like to bring you into still deeper waters where the footing is not so secure, nor the catch so certain. I would ask your attention to the relations between Psychopathology and what is known as " Organic Disease."

In order to prepare the way, permit me to take you back to the beginning of things and by a series of lantern slides develop a concept of the human machine which will, I hope, give you something to bite on even if it threatens to dislocate any but the most solid of jaws.

I shall avoid the more heavy scholastic repetition of what should be well known ideas, how for instance, Descartes (1596–1650) and de la Mettrie developed the idea of man as a machine, nor shall I weary you with the mumbo-jumbo of the philosophers and metaphysicians who have squabbled and will continue so to do over mechanistic and vitalistic antagonistic hypothese, nor with that equally threadbare controversial topic of the relationship of body and/or mind.

Although we shall lean fairly heavily on general mechanistic con-

* Read as part of a symposium at the Annual Meeting of the Medical Society of the State of New York, at Syracuse, N. Y., June 2, 1931. Courtesy of *New York State Jl. Medicine,* 32, 1932, 581, May 15.

ceptions I would in more simple terms emphasize the fact that Man is not a " Jack in the Box." Practically every activity that goes on in man is infinitely more subtle and complex than what we at the present time understand. And the reason is obvious if we only stop a moment to think about man as a time-binding animal. Although we glibly use the terms " heredity " and " constitution " it is but rarely that we realize how long this heaping up of the past upon the past has been going on and just what has been happening in the gradual evolutionary ascent from Amoeba to Man in the billion years that it took to have this goal of Man reached.

I like to recall the term that Samuel Butler used about this process by which all experience in time became bound up in bodily structures. He called it " Organic Memory." And if you would ask for a clue as to who had worked up this set of problems most consecutively I would refer you to the works of Hering, and more particularly to those of Semon, starting with his celebrated study on the " Mneme." Should we but stop to imagine what this mnemic inheritance really means the stoutest of us would be staggered. Should I by way of an interpolation state that at times certain individuals suffer from what I shall provisionally call " total recall " of much of these memory traces, *i.e.,* are unable to keep them from pressing over the portals of consciousness, such patients we speak of as psychotic, as in delirium or in manic-stuporous states, for instance, and we can well understand why in times, not too long gone by, so many of them have been spoken of as " possessed."

Thus I would call your specific attention to at least two important preliminary considerations; namely, that accumulation of organic memories of billions of years in the making and which we will speak of as the " wisdom of the body," and those devices which have arisen to bind, inhibit, or repress organic processes from expressing themselves as simply as does the " Jack in the Box " with which figure I began this paragraph.

Just what these protective devices of physico-chemical binding, or physiological inhibition and of psychological repression are, will occupy us later after attention is called to a schematic representation of the energic hypothesis—grossly mechanistic if you will—whereby the human being as well as all living organisms may be conceived of as capturing, transforming and delivering the energy of the cosmos of which they are an integral part. Man and his environment are one. He is not an independent isolated experience. He exists only by reason of and through this interchange of activities between his organic processes which his organic memory of how to handle them has, when successful, enabled him to live.

The figure 1 before you roughly indicates this situation.   It is unnecessary for me to go into the details of the receptors which capture the energy any more than by saying that the kindergarten physiologies that speak of five senses must be relegated to oblivion. We have twenty and more definitely structuralized sensory receptors. Different types exist in every organ of the body and through the

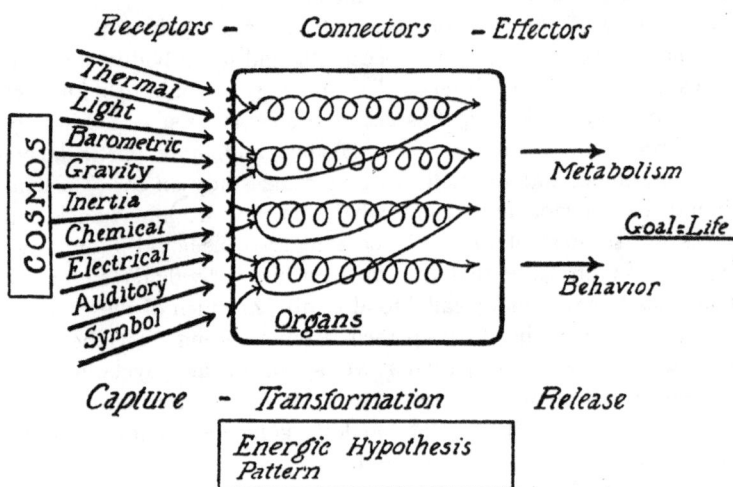

FIGURE 1

medium of a most highly complex switchboard series of nerve-net transformers all the literally billions of outside calls are handled by automatic processes.   Here in the diagram may be seen a thumb-nail sketch of physiology whereby and through which all the incoming experience becomes converted into processes of upkeep of the machine (anabolism and catabolism) and of the individual in society (behavior).

The moment one attempts to follow through any one of the incoming bits of cosmic reality—let us say a vestibular or an auditory stimulus we are into the thick of details of histological receptor, and physiological transmitter and connector complexities, the study of any one or the other of which some men devote an entire life to; as

Helmholtz for instance did for the optical apparatus. I can refer you to no better guide of these complexities than C. Winkler's Manual of Neurology.

What does our "bodily wisdom" do with the billions of stimuli after they all stream in? Like any other billion year old factory which has been more and more successfully operated would do it has *organized* its responses, or if you will, they have organized themselves, and as in the next diagram certain patterns of performance have evolved. It is not of much particular moment what one calls these patterns; it is only desirable that in giving them a shorthand name, man should come to some sort of agreement as to what the name should stand for. Up to the present time biology has fairly

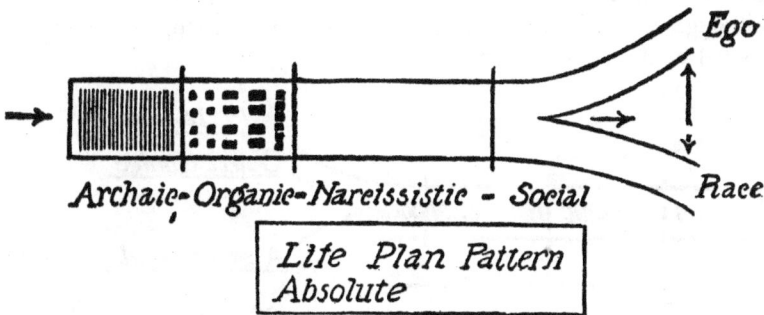

FIGURE 2

well agreed, not without, of course, the usual clash of opinions about everything, to call the outstanding patterns of response to these processes of capturing, transforming and delivering the cosmic energy— "instinct patterns." Without going into the numerous objections we will follow this lead and for all types of living things, plant and animal, distinguish two instinct patterns which have come to be called that of Self-Preservation and that of Race Propagation. Schiller, the poet, it will be recalled, termed them "Hunger and Love." While there has been and still is much dispute, filling millions of books, as to the comparative importance and significance of these two patterns I shall arbitrarily state that the creative, race-propagation pattern is the one which fundamentally must lead else there would have been no such thing as the evolution of new types of structure from Amoeba to Man. A moment's reflection will show this is obvious, although thousands of books are written about the more intimate details of the conflicting claims between the " self " and the " race." The slogan that " self-preservation is the first law of nature " is one of those universally shouted slogans which like most universal slogans are usually wrong. A great philosopher has been quoted for nineteen centuries—" he who would save his life must lose it." Even though this quotation is rarely thought of as contributing to the significance of the conception that the race-propagation instinct pattern is the one that has the " beat " in life's flow from form to form, nevertheless this is what it signifies.

This leads to the next diagram (Fig. 3) that would dissect this internal pattern of striving or impulse, or urge, or drive, or any other synonym that one wishes, a little more in order to bring it into some objective form. All of this is still in the " wisdom of the body " although we are now coming a bit more into the open out of the tunnel of the unknown past.

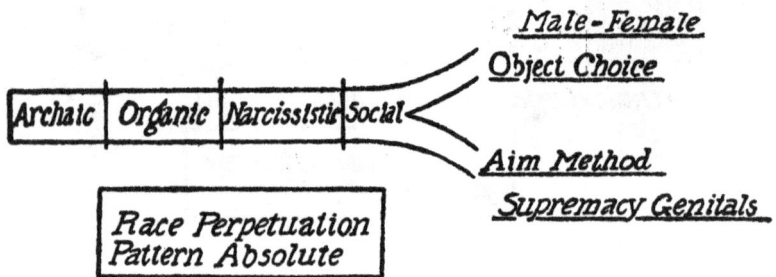

FIGURE 3

In short no such thing as reproduction is going to take place, at the biological level, unless a union takes place between differentiated carriers of life's experience, termed respectively male and female. Some " ninnies," I call them, meaning no offense, set up a great to do as to the comparative values of male and female in this respect. At the biological level this is hokum. As no lock operates (rightly) without a key, so no key is any good except for a lock and so it goes— male and female are like our previous pair, individual and environment. If the latter is out of gear—life is impossible; if the former— continuance of life in new forms is impossible. The exceptional forms of repetition through fission as in bacteria, potatoes or lily bulbs, are of no moment at this juncture.

And as our diagram further shows—that unless male spermatozoon, through penis-vagina transmission, fertilizes female ova, no new form results. This is again so obvious as to almost make one naïve in saying it and yet an important principle is here involved. As all of you here know that when the urge, or drive or impulse—originally named after the god Eros—sometimes misses its object-choice (male-female) and/or its aim (penis-vagina) there results those anomalies of behavior described in the large chapter of sociological pathology of the inversions and the perversions.

This leads to the first large generalization about pattern activities which I shall emphasize as of paramount significance if we are ever going to understand the relations of psychopathology to organic disease.

This is that: *Any deviation from object or aim threatens the harmonious action patterns within the machine.*

There's a catch somewhere in this simple statement. It is literally true but needs an important emphasis to be put upon those aspects of man's impulses, drives, urges or what have you, of which man is not aware—that is within his *Unconscious.* We are not here concerned in this formulation with the individual's conscious notions concerning his object choice or his aims, although such may be in line with the vastly more important automatic unconscious processes of the wisdom of the body of which mention has been made.

An ancient prophet once wrote "All men are liars." In these matters psychoanalytic science prefers to use a more careful term. It says " all men rationalize." They have the tendency to make their belief agreeable ; as out of the fullness of the heart the mouth speaketh, so most of our explanations of our pattern motivation is autistic— *i.e.,* wish fulfilling. Here is the catch that is necessary to understand if one would comprehend what part is played in the entire picture that may be termed psychological, or psychic, or what Socrates called the soul. We will not split hairs just now about these similar and differing conceptions.

If our original postulate be correct that man is a billion year time-bound series of structuralized experiences with Nature then it can be understood that the vast majority of his activities take place absolutely beyond his knowledge, *i.e.,* beyond his conscious perceptions. Attention has been called to the chemical bindings, reflex inhibitions and reflexes and psychological repressions that protect him from instant response to all of the stimuli about him, and which if such traps or devices were not there would reduce him, as sometimes does happen, to that situation of the humorist who would ask, " What happens if a chameleon be placed upon a Scotch plaid? " Out of this we emerge with a statement cast in the form of a proportion.

As from minute to minute is to a billion years so are our Conscious reasons for doing things to the " Unconscious " processes that really bring them about.

This means then an entirely new technique has to be employed to get at the truth locked up in the wisdom of the body, *i.e.,* the " Unconscious." Before entering into this new technique, as a technique, let me briefly outline what it has seemed to teach us and I do so in the next diagram which would offer a picture of our mental systems. This is slightly modified, for our purposes, from the ideas that Freud has conceived. This egg-shaped figure (Figure 4) may be said to represent three essential parts of our mental systems.

During the billion years of accumulation of experience there was fashioned a vast variety of automatic responses to Nature's stimuli to which the general term, the Id, might be applied. All forms of life have a psychic life, for by psychic we would here mean *total response,* or purposeful pattern action. In higher forms there developed out of the Id a perceptive system which became what we call " conscious " when by reason of environmental fluctuations automatic adaptive action was faulty. Such fluctuations needed quick sizing up in order to alter older structural repetitive habitual actions. To that part of the Id which was in conscious touch with reality as a tester, Freud, in his metapsychology, gave the name of " Ego." This " Ego " must not be confused with the popular term " ego " which more properly is termed the Self—or for myself I prefer the term the " M-ego."

An outstanding function of this part of the mental system, the Ego is to suppress and to repress the urges, or impulses, or action patterns of the Id which would be disadvantageous to the self, the individual, or to society. We speak of them popularly as self-control, judgment, reason, logic, etc., etc. Through the study of science has come the richest store for this guiding instrument of the Ego to suppress consciously and repress unconsciously powerful Id forces.

As Freud studied dreams carefully he noted an extremely interesting series of phenomena such as a chemist might, by analogy, note in the process of fractional distillation or its reverse. He saw that another system was at work changing the crude Id symbols, fractionating them so that they could come to some form of expression acceptable to the individual's Ego. He called this "Censorship" and it too was of the nature of repression—not "Censor" as has

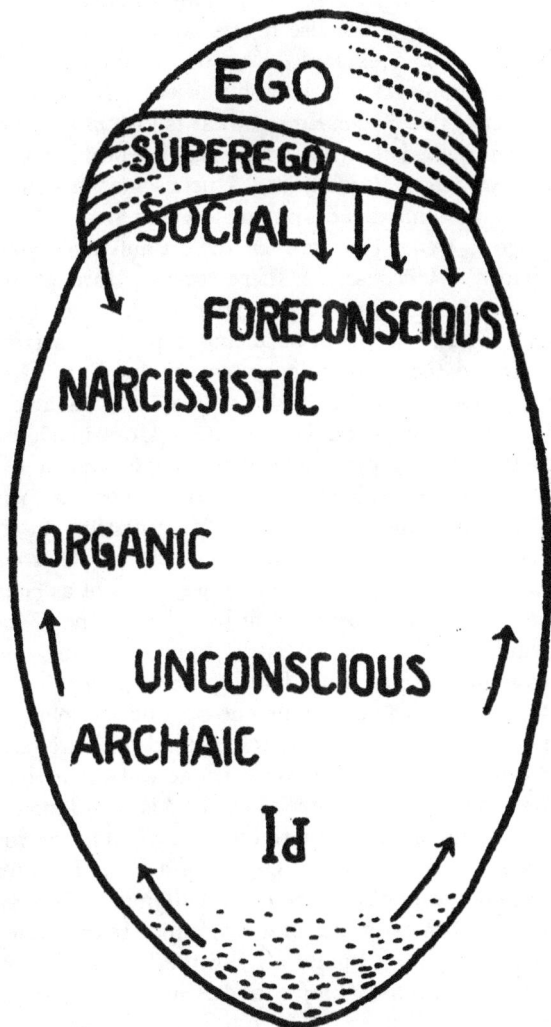

Figure 4

Purely schematic diagram of the arrangement of the mental apparatus. Physical-chemical-biological experiences and impulses operating as primitive Id forces—controlled for socialized expression (creative libido) by inhibiting, repressing, and suppressing forces of the Ego and Super-Ego.

been so widely written. It is a term for a dynamic "process."
Further consideration led Freud—and I speak very, very briefly here
of this highly important part of the mental systems—to call this the
Ego-Ideal or Super-Ego, because it was largely built up from childhood upon precept and example—*i.e.*, upon authority, first of the
father and mother images and later by others. In the popular par-
lance one aspect of this Super-Ego is what is known as "conscience."
It is somewhat related to what some people speak of as intuition.
Dr. Brill has written of it partly as "Unconscious Insight."

Consider for a moment the diagram—where it will be noted that
the Super-Ego is wedged in between the Id and the Ego—one part
in contact with the Unconscious, there reaching through the preconscious or foreconscious and at its upper level in contact with the
"Conscious." Here is a sort of balancing, repressing system working
as an auxiliary to the repressing system of the Ego. It is certain
that certain processes in the "Id" will always be inaccessible to
conscious control: repression is absolute. How much no one yet
knows and this is of great importance to the student of so-called
organic disease processes. That which from moment to moment is
held under by repression but may be made accessible by effort or by
other factors is the *foreconscious or preconscious:* That which occu-
pies, as it were, the center of awareness we speak of as *conscious.* It
will be seen that Freud's formulation here is not one of location but
one of dynamics. There is no such thing as *in* the unconscious;
unconscious mind, etc.; such are faulty phrasings of this general conception. If to use a chemical simile one says that gasoline is "unconscious" in crude oil, but by a definite heat and pressure technique can
be isolated out, *i.e.,* be made conscious, one can get a rough idea of
how these terms are understood. The "Id" is the crude oil. Should
I change my metaphor to one more mechanical and very rough, think
of a running internal-cumbustion engine of a Rolls-Royce car turned
out after a billion years of experience in building. The motive power
comes from the Cosmos of our first diagram. It runs day and night
and is always on its way (Immortality of the Race). Its goal is some
definite place and purpose (Object and Aim). Its patterns of action
are the roads that lead there. The Ego in our scheme is the steering
gear and the gas feed. The Super-Ego—the hand and foot brake.
If one is perfectly clear as to the place and the road, one needs but to
step on the gas and steer with judgment, ever alert for some variable
in the environment to automatically shut off the gas or suddenly to

put on the foot brake or if needs be suppress and repress all movement by the hand brake. The human motor only stalls with death.

Why is all this complicated series of dynamics necessary? Because
from the cradle to the grave some parts of the mental systems are
called into action. In childhood the Id forces are all powerful and
the Ego is weak. The care of authority, the " Super-Ego," is necessary. Here is where religion has been of so much value in the
gradual development of man from the primitive to the present.

For the weaker the Ego, as with the infant, the greater must be the
parental care for the individual. In a civilized community the State
must play a similar rôle. For the weaker the Ego the greater the
Fear needed to control, hence at the lower levels of the Super-Ego
one finds magic, superstition, ritualistic observances, etc. As the
Ego grows and begins to understand physical and chemical
realities the needs for authority outside become less and less and little
by little the creative and destructive forces of the Id are subjected
to greater conscious control.

In diagram 2 the life pattern was roughly divided into four stages.
We might have been Shakespearean and made seven but four are
sufficiently illustrative of the general idea. In the Archaic period
(intrauterne), the libido is actively creating organs to fulfill the
ancestral hereditary patterns in structure and function. In the nine
months the libido has rapidly recapitulated the ascent of life from
protozoon to mammal. A piteous, helpless animal at birth, but with
a richer heritage behind it than before it. In the next seven years,
to relapse to Shakespeare's numbers, the adaptive harmony of the
organ needs is to be established. Here environmental forces are more
variable than in the intrauterine bath. There is great rivalry among
these various organs. Each seeks its own functional satisfactions by
obtaining pleasure and avoiding pain by hook or crook or by the
reality or the phantasy pathways. It is to this period that search will
have to be directed for the roots of those organic disorders with which
psychopathology may be concerned. As the personality enters into
the conscious stage, " Cogito-ergo-sum " of Descartes, the individual
enters a " Narcissistic " stage! " Papa look "—" Mama look ";
" everybody look at *me* "; " at *my* this and that "! The libido Id
strivings having obtained a fair degree of organ satisfaction now is
focussed on the entire Myself, the " M-ego." " I love me " is the
keynote of this, roughly speaking seven- to fourteen-year-old developmental stage during which certain organ supremacy of striving is

maturing. Then man enters the puberty period and his greatest shove forward towards " Id " impulse gratification takes place. With the exception of his Ego organ—the brain chiefly—all of his organs are as mature as they are going to be, speaking generally and for the average. It is at this period that a great deal of personality break-down takes place for which Morel, the penetrating French psychia-trist, coined the expression—" stranded on the rock of puberty " and which marks the period when personality development is subjected

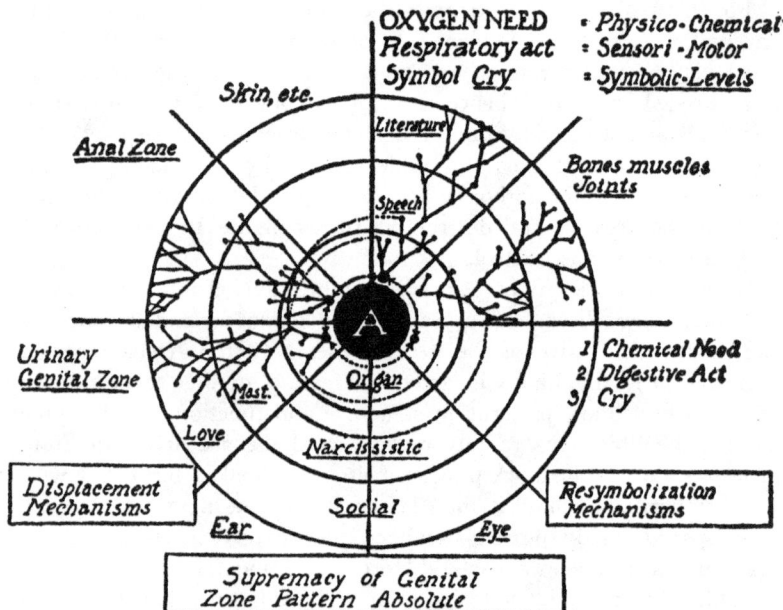

Figure 5

to the greatest whirlwinds of environmental stress because of the force of the Id impulses. Here is where a well-balanced Super-Ego, from successfully adapted parents plays an important rôle and when ignorant, bigoted and malignant forces of magic, superstition, and false authority of education, religion or social activities start conflicts within the mental systems which augur ill for the developing individual.

Two *concurrent* trends of action patterns have been maturing throughout these four stages. In Figure 5 is roughly shown the evolution from the infantile to adult organ libido utilization. At first the child lives only to breathe (and holler), then to eat (and swallow), then to urinate and then to defecate. Here prudery "*a la* Comstock, Sumner and Co.*"* suggests Latin terms for the latter two homely words of repressed or suppressed enjoyment. The Latin takes the fun out but admits a wider expression of gratification. What one loses thereby in quality perhaps is evened up in quantity, this sort of balancing between primitive joys with their more austere social permissions in modified form is the great work of the Super-Ego and Ego inhibiting and repressing systems. Thus by way of crude illustration one may say that the primitive joy of working over one's feces in the colon may be sublimated in the activities of the sculptor or dabbler in oils and paints. The plumber, hydraulic engineer or creator of " Muscle Shoals " works out to varying degrees of complete mastery the omnipotence that once gripped the bladder and started it on its pattern of eons of preparation. I might, had I the time and you the endurance, trace out from the acorn of every organ's mastery of its destiny to the oak of its ultimate supremacy in the orderly socialized distribution of the titanic forces that reside in the Id of Everyman.

Of one special chapter in this evolution, that of the " supremacy of the genital " functioning, millions of words might be spoken and none ever the same that would trace the nascent impulses through organic growth, through adolescent self love, to object love and finally to the building of those values of the most supreme achievement in human society. If to that force the word " Libido " be attached I would remind you of its far reaching importance in every bit of living endeavor.

And finally to my last diagram which would seek to illustrate what Freud has called the " nuclear " complex in the human libido distribution, patterning it after the intuitive insight of Sophocles' tragic drama of King Œdipus. Were you to come with me into any one of our state hospitals, you would very soon be amazed at the frank expressions of the Œdipus situation from numerous patients. As I have previously reminded you many of these patients are suffering from varying degrees of " total recall." The past of the " Id " breaks through the repressions of both Ego and Super-Ego and the faint or stark skeletons of the Œdipus nucleus stand forth. Like Mark Twain's celebrated story of how human speech at the North Pole became frozen and then thawed out in a claque of strange sounds as the temperature became warmer, so the repressed material breaking through gives one a superior insight into " what every one of us is dragging behind him unawares."

The pathway taken by the libido in its developmental investments of objects away from those of the uterus, the cradle, the kindergarten, away from infantile bladder, or bowel, or muscular, or skin pleasure—pain attachment to identifications of mother (pleasure principle) or father (reality principle) is roughly sketched in these two diagrams.

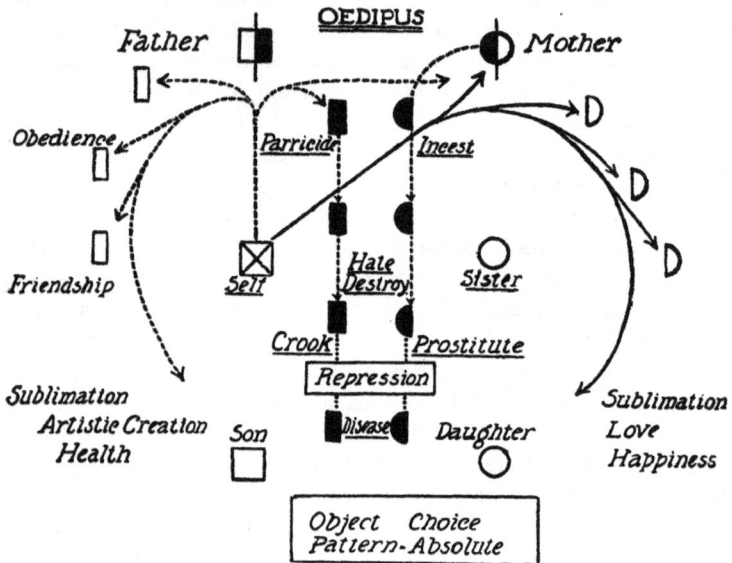

FIGURE 6

And this leads to the final statement and explanation of what is involved when certain types of organic disease are being dissected psychologically to endeavor to find the deviation from Object and Aim in the libido strivings.

To understand this attention might first be called to the universal mechanism of *Conversion* that mankind uses to as it were " pass the buck " to his Ego by paying penance to his Super-Ego.

In its mildest forms it is seen behind the innumerable ready excuses that one gives when one would avoid something. Such are the innumerable make-believe " headaches " and " fatigue states " to get out of doing something and to continue doing something more desired. More heavily loaded conflicts bring about, not these semi-conscious subterfuges, but repression, which pushing more strongly throws the conflict into the Unconscious. The Id, however, always demands expression and the Super-Ego takes hold of it and says, "Yes, you can have it but it will hurt you." Here the hysteria conversion mechanism is in evidence. The punishment penance paid to the Super-Ego blinds the Ego as to the real significance of the Id craving and so one has the innumerable kinds of bodily "organ neuroses" with which the hysteria literature is full. Now only one step further is needed to convert a benign reversible conversion process which is called hysteria into a malignant conversion process which can make an "organ neurosis" over into an irreversible organic disease, when, for instance, a grasping, impatient stomach develops its peptic ulcer or an intestine its duodenal ulcer.

The one step further is simply a question as to the amount of libido investment that is frozen in a fixation at an organ erotic level and its persistence. I need hardly remind you how a frozen investment can upset one's financial adaptation after October, 1929's, experience. The hysterical non-malignant conversion outbreak is a safety valve, a defense reaction against either specific local social environmental hardships or against discomforts of civilization at a more general level.

Finally I would show in diagrammatic form a rough outline of how a chronic malignant conversion might take the form of a hypertensive nephrosis. It could occupy me many hours discussing this one of similar mechanisms some of which I have put in print as have Groddeck, Deutsch, Allendy and others since my initial contribution to this type of problem in 1916.

Very briefly a distracted husband came to me demanding I save his wife. The doctors, he said, gave her six months to live. She had Brights disease and needed a diet and rest in bed or she would die. It is no great news to you to be told that some of us are a bit pessimistic and alarmists and I told him so and to calm down and tell me the story. Here it is on the chart. (See Figure 7 on page 22.)

I told him I had not treated kidney disease for many years but I would send her to the best hospital I knew and take her over the works and then translate to his engineering mind the verbalizations of the internists. They practically said "she had high blood pressure because she had kidney disease and kidney disease because she had high blood pressure." Being an engineer this did not go far with him, nor her as far as that goes, and I agreed to do a little exploration of the "Unconscious" in the terms here already briefly sketched.

A woman, aged 36, married, children ♀, ♂, ♀, ♀, nephritis-hypertension.

Symptoms

Headache four years. Blood pressure 240-250 mm. Albumin. Diminished urea output. Retention. Asthenia. Edema. Dyspnea. Constipation + + +. Slight momentary lapses.

Behavior

Able, energetic, cultivated interests in home, children, society. Two girls in family. Devoted father; beautiful, much admired mother. Large family group of professional people. Never peculiar. No eccentricities.

Unconscious

Oedipus evolutions, defective. Strong father fixation. Rejection of male. Homophilic. Supremacy of genital zone, defective. Urinary fixations. Strong anal erotic components.

FIGURE 7

Chart of symptoms of the case.

And since the dream is the royal road into the Unconscious my exploration began with the dream, the first one of which, she recalled while in the hospital was as follows:

It was in the country somewhere, a path led from a house to a country road. Coming from right to left, at a lickety-split rate of speed, were two men in racing sulkies. As they swept by in a cloud of dust, a woman ran out of the house towards them with disheveled hair and apparently shrieking to stop—or what, she was not sure. They went on their way up a steep hill without slackening their pace and when they got to the top one turned to the left and ran into a stone wall two feet high and smashed horse and sulky and everything to pieces.

" Well," I said, " a cheerful picture; and suppose you did a thing like that what would you think about it? "

" What do you mean? " she replied.

" Well," I said, " an ancient Greek philosopher, Heraklitus, once said something like this. This was 500 B.C. and long before Freud: ' For the waking there is one common world; but for those asleep, each one turns aside to his own privacy.' And do you imagine you could do with impunity what you dream? Is it not because you lie still and do not act that you can indulge your fancies?"

"Well," she said slowly, "one would be crazy to do a thing like that such as in the dream."

"Good," I said, "let us see wherein there is a crazy drive that is destroying you." Here, you see, there is a different method of approach than the blood pressure—kidney disease—dog-chasing-his-tail mode of explanation.

In the methodology of psychoanalysis it was very soon obvious wherein this woman was out of line with the inner laws of nature. She was at odds with her own instinctive patterns. The race instinct pattern was all wrong. In spite of the fact that she had had four children she had been frigid. Even clitoris manipulation left her cold. Her organ erotic fixation was even more primitive than that, it was urethral. She got her supreme gratification at that level. She urinated quarts to get it, and drank gallons to get the quarts, and in a-b-c short order, the heart, the blood vessels and finally the kidney had to hand it along in double time and finally rebelled. This is not the whole story. It is only a glimpse at the main issues. It would take many hours for me to outline to your or my satisfaction how this particular mode of organ outlet finally was chosen and what was the significance of early identifications and what were the patterns taken up into her "Super-Ego." And how this failure of the Super-Ego to work with the Ego and the "Id" destroyed her, just as she had destroyed the man (her father) in the racing sulky in her dream.

When the ancient psalmist said, "Vengeance is mine, I shall repay, saith the Lord," he was only saying in an intuitive lingo what the ancient dramatists said when they talked about Fate, and what the modern scientific imagination calls the study of the immutable laws of nature. When we refuse to get in line with nature, as registered in the faulty purposes of life—i.e., our mental states—even the kidneys, the blood pressure and urea, proteid, ionic milieu become involved and this is but one formula for many diseases.

She did not die in six months—she lived eight years of a useful, busy life, and only went to bed in the last month of her life. Innumerable details of what psychotherapy did to her blood pressure and her kidney states might be detailed here. I might even be able to show how she escaped from the vigilance of the Ego and finally how the Super-Ego forced the punishment of death. But this would be a long, long story.

NOTE

(Dr. Jelliffe then demonstrated lantern slides with explanatory remarks of the malignant formation of a bony tumor, the development of oculogyric crises in post-encephalitic states, a chronic esophageal diverticulum case that developed a psychosis when operation cured the diverticulum, a case of duodenal ulcer of psychogenic causation and an interesting chronic dyspepsia with rumination and cardiospasm which was traced back to the infant's mastery over her mother when at the breast. Some of these cases have been reported more fully in special articles. See Bibliography.)

BIBLIOGRAPHY (Partial Only)

DEUTSCH, F.: Psychoanalyse und Organkrankheiten, *Zeit. Psa.*, 8, 290, 1922. Die Bedeutung psychoanalytischer Kenntnisse für die innere Medizin, *Mitt. d. Grenz. inn. Med. u. Khk.*, 21, 1, 1922. Ueber die Bildung Conversions Symptoms, *Zeit. Psa.*, 8, 480, 1922, ib. 10, 380, 1924; 12, 493, 1916.

FERENCZI, S.: Diseases or Patho-Neuroses. Further Contributions. Hogarth Press, London, 1926.

FREUD, S.: Gesammlte Schriften.

GRODDECK, G.: The Book of the It, Nervous and Mental Disease Publishing Co., New York and Washington. Our Unknown Selves, Daniels, London: Die psychische Bedingtheit und psychoanalytische Behandlung organischer Leiden, Hirzel, 1917. Eine Symptom Analyse, *Zeit. Psa.*, 6, 320, 1920. Ueber die psychoanalytischer Behandlung organischer Krankheiten, *Zeit. Psa.*, 7, 252, 1920.

JELLIFFE, S. E., and WHITE, W. A.: Diseases of the Nervous System, 5th Ed., 1929, Lea & Febiger, Philadelphia. Psoriasis as a Conversion Symptom, *N. Y. Med. Jl.*, Dec., 1916. Epileptic Attack in Dynamic Pathology, *N. Y. Med. Jl.*, July 27, 1918. Psychotherapy and Tuberculosis, *Am. Jl. Tb.*, 3, 417, 1919. Multiple Sclerosis and Psychoanalysis, *Am. Jl. M. Sc.*, 161, 666, 1921; *J. N. M. Dis.*, May, 1922. Psychopathology and Organic Disease, *Arch. Neur. & Psych.*, 8, 639, 1922. Neuropathology and Bone Disease, *Tr. Am. Neur. Assoc.*, 1923, 419. Old Age Factor in Psychoanalytic Therapy, *Med. Jl. & Record*, 1925, 121. Unconscious Dynamics and Human Behavior, Prince Memorial, Harcourt, Brace, N. Y., 1925. Psychoanalysis and Organic Disorder; Myopia, *Int. Jl. Psa.*, 7, 445, 1926. Post-encephalitic Respiratory Disorders, Nerv. & Ment. Dis. Monographs, 1927. Hysteria, Osler Mod. Med., 3rd Edit., 1928. Postencephalitic Oculogyric Crises, *Arch. Neur. & Psych.*, 21, 491, 1929; 23, 1227, 1930; *J. N. & Dis.*, 69, 59 *et seq.*, 1929. Diencephalitic Vegetative Mechanisms, *Arch. Neur. & Psych.*, 21, 838, 1929. What Price Healing, *J. A. M. A.*, 94, 1393, 1930. *Vigilance, Psa. Rev.*, 17, 305, 1930. Dupuytren's Contracture and the Unconscious, *Int. Clinics*, 41, Ser. III, 184, 1931.

III.

THE DEATH INSTINCT IN SOMATIC PATHOLOGY AND PSYCHOPATHOLOGY *

And if to some my tale seems foolishness
I am content that such could count me fool.
Sophocles: Oedipus in Coloneus.

In my early thirties, while I was still in the beginnings of my medical career and was trying to earn an honest penny by work outside of the actual practice of medicine, I became editor of the *Medical News,* then one of the oldest of the medical weeklies of the United States.

The annual meetings of the American Medical Association were events of much moment to editors of the four or five medical weeklies then existing, and hence I attended them. In 1904, the annual meeting was held at Portland, Oregon, and it was at that time that an occasion was offered to visit Alaska, and I traveled as far north as the great divide, down which the gold rush descended in that memorable push to the golden sands of the Yukon.

One of the strange events of this trip which burned in my memory at that time, and which constitutes the beginning of this contribution was the vivid picture of the mad climb of the salmon up the rivers of the western coast, carrying out their strange and fatal journey during which the instinctual impulses of life and death fought out their implicit patterns in grotesque antithesis.

If ever the lines " In the midst of life we are in death," which came as a faint echo from an earlier period of my life, were obscure in my mind as to explicit meaning, here there was no doubt that such a paradox was patent as well as potent.

It was not by any means the first time that the phenomenon in question had come to my notice. As one interested in natural history it was an old story, and here might well provide an essay, but not until I actually saw the billions of salmon caught in the grip of the death instinct after their frantic struggle to carry out the work of Eros did the whole adventure possess any vivid reality. Nor did it

* Reprinted by permission from the *Transactions of the American Neurological Association,* 1932.

25

seem to have any intimate relation with human life apart from the mystic words of religious construction until the fertilizing thoughts of Freud gave new meanings for many of the problems of medicine.

When nearly twenty years later I first read Freud's "Beyond the Pleasure Principle" (1920) and, later, his "Ego and the Id" (1923), the whole series of conceptions connected with the strange behavior of the salmon was reëvoked.

Even as a youth I realized that at moments there came to every one the wish to die. I had read about it in books, and some of my most striking experiences in my ambulance activities were of suicide. Later, as a psychiatrist, melancholia and the manic-depressive cycle intrigued my curiosity; this was all to little avail until the connecting links between the mad maniacal climb-urge of mania and the sad retreat of melancholia as a following out of the principle of the conflict of the life and death instincts were made by Freud.

Then came a long period of close and intense analytic work with partial and localized forms of this instinctual defusion in so-called organic disease.

It had been a commonplace observation to note a frank psychotic expression of conflict clear up and to find as an alternative in the same patient a disturbance of renal function, a marked skin disorder, diabetes or a hyperthyroid state. In a number of cyclothymic persons there was observed a regular replacement of the one group of manifestations by the other. When the neurotic or psychotic manifestations were in the ascendancy, the anomalous somatic behavior sank beneath the horizon, to emerge into a definite form as the more evident "mental" expressions in their turn faded out of the picture. And thus the replacement cycle went on.

Finally the generalization became more clear as the conception of the holistic nature of man became more evident; the human being as a whole was seen in a constant state of unstable equilbrium, and further, functional variability as evidence of the struggle of energy systems within and without the body was the rule rather than the exception.

Medical science in the past century has opened up a clearer vision of those energy systems from both without (trauma-infection) and within (metabolic), but it was not until the genius of Freud developed a similar unitary understanding of the dynamics (economics) of the mental systems from *without* (as bound up in customs, folklore, religions, caste and class) and from *within* (such as identification with parents, Œdipus structural patterns, and instinct drives) that a true holistic view of many disease processes could be gained.

It was then that the mental or psychologic or (purposeful meaning) component to be found in practically all disease processes became a burning subject of inquiry. I then began to study certain chronic maladies, such as skin diseases (eczema and psoriasis[1]), lung disease (asthma, chronic bronchitis and tuberculosis[2]), kidney disease (hypertension nephroses[3] and tubercle of kidney), bone and joint disease (bony tumors,[4] arthritides and contractures[5]), spinal cord disease,[6] thyroid imbalance[7] and eye disorders (myopia[8]), with the object in view of trying to separate out the conflict of the life and death instinctual processes that finally became encysted or segregated in an organ or organs where the fight was carried out either as a temporary moratorium or in the form of a final adjustment of claims, with partial or complete destruction of the organ unconsciously chosen as a site for the conflict.

Some of these observations have found their way into print as more or less definite forms of expression. None of these expositions has been entirely satisfactory, for obvious reason. One would require a book really to satisfy all of the various issues that arise in trying to elaborate the successive steps in the psychobiologic processes involved in even the simplest of the compromise formations (diseases as "scapegoats") here envisaged (certain dermatoses for instance).

Much as I might like to comfort myself with the thought that the presentation of these analyses has been incomplete and unsatisfactory because of difficulties surrounding or bound up in all psychoanalytic

---

[1] Jelliffe, S. E.: Psoriasis as an Hysterical Conversion Symptom. *New York M. J.*, 104 : 1077, 1916.

[2] Jelliffe, S. E., and Evans, E.: Psychotherapy and Tuberculosis. *Am. Rev. Tuberc.*, 3 : 417, 1919.

[3] Jelliffe, S. E.: Psychopathology and Organic Disease. *Arch. Neurol. & Psychiat.*, 8 : 639 (Dec.), 1922.

[4] Jelliffe, S. E.: Neuropathology and Bone Disease. *Tr. Am. Neurol A.*, 1923, p. 419.

[5] Jelliffe, S. E.: Dupuytren's Contracture and the Unconscious. *Internat. Clin.*, 3 : 184 (Sept.), 1931.

[6] Jelliffe, S. E.: Multiple Sclerosis, the Vegetative Nervous System and Psychoanalytic Research. *Arch. Neurol. & Psychiat.*, 4 : 593 (Nov.), 1920; *Am. J. M. Sc.*, 161 : 666, 1921; *J. Nerv. & Ment. Dis.*, 55 : 309, 1922.

[7] Jellffe, S. E.: The Psyche and the Vegetative Nervous System, with Special Reference to Some Endocrinopathies. *New York M. J.*, 115 : 382, 1922.

[8] Jelliffe, S. E.: Psychoanalyse und organische Störung: Myopie als Paradigma. *Internat. Ztschr. f. Psychoanal.*, 12 : 517, 1926; translated in *Internat. J. Psycho-Analysis*, 7 : 445, 1926.

case histories, some factors of which, medical secrecy for instance, are of major significance, I must regretfully acknowledge that the carrying through of the theoretical considerations necessary for real proof has been far from satisfactory, especially when I look back on the work of analysis, in which I have been late in grasping a truer significance of many situations with that firmness which later experience has permitted.[9]

Above all it might be recalled that the human machine is no simple " Jack-in-the-Box." As it takes great patience to dissect persistently the complex and subtle psychic processes, infinitely more compounded than any other in human activities, so it would require volumes of the words and concepts now available to report such micropsychic dissections. It is revealing that Freud in his " Fragment," as he calls it, of an analysis of a case of hysteria fills 146 large octavo pages, in English translation, and in my opinion there is not a useless or redundant phrase in this whole presentation.

The point to be emphasized about these personal studies has been that the sadistic (hostility) component (death instinct) has operated as a castration or partial death of an organ or of certain functions of an organ and thus brought about the disharmony of function. In some instances it has been more malignant (irreversible) than in others. I have therefore subsumed them more clearly as instances of malignant conversion (irreversible processes) in which the conversion mechanism as such, follows, in part, those seen in the less malignant hysterias (reversible processes). The quantitative factors which have interfered with an adequate compromise of the conflict can be envisaged chiefly through the conception of the *tyranny* of the Super-Ego mechanism. The law of retribution, *lex talionis,* has been too rigorously carried out. Just how this comes to be, chiefly because of the libido regression being fixated in early organic erotic stages, hence involving adjuvant instinctual frustration, cannot be further elaborated in this paper.

In one of my reported cases, a definite adolescent myopia [8] could be demonstrated (to my satisfaction at least) as a classic illustration of such a type of castration punishment for infantile peeping, prying crimes carried out at primitive fixated levels involving the unsublimated remnants of the Œdipus complex.

It is not my intention at this time to attempt to generalize on these various observations in different indicated fields or to follow along

[9] Freud, S.: The Ego and the Id. London: Hogarth Press, 1928.

the same pathways with newer ones, although in my daily work such material is steadily accumulating.

In the present communication, I wish to reverse the whole story and to attempt to present an idea looking toward an understanding of how certain procedures which are in widespread use in the treatment of certain mental conditions can be thought of as accomplishing some of their beneficial results in accordance with certain aspects of meaning which constitute a mirror picture of the preceding considerations. Such a presentation seems not inapproprate historically at this centenary of "Alice in Wonderland," "Alice in the Looking Glass," classics.

In order to do this I should like first to review briefly some of the freudian conceptions which bear on the idea to be presented.

As one traces instinctual processes back to their origins one inevitably turns up the work of the sexual impulse, the work of Eros as Freud has aptly termed it. " The clamor of life proceeds for the most part from Eros." Sadistic or destructive components (death instincts—Thanatos) are always fused with Eros, but are usually " mute." In the melancholias we know they " speak," and they also speak quite volubly in the so-called " paranoias," " compulsion neuroses " in which last types they show all of the destructive tendencies behind all fanatic ceremonial. Such fixed ceremonials are exemplified in history in the story of the *sense of guilt and the need for punishment* from the time of the history of the " expulsion from the garden of Eden " to the present day, with Calvin and the execution of Michel Servetus, the Inquisition and the burning of witches, as prominent replicas in the middle foreground. This voice of Thanatos, that is, sadism, which operates chiefly, though not exclusively, through the repressions of the Super-Ego (conscience in part) often does not break through into the conscious Ego system as the pain of depression or of phobies, as compulsions, as conversions or as projections in hallucinatory or delusional formations, all of which have come to be evolved economically as *saviors of the organs* of the body.

When a complete release of all of the sexual tensions from top to bottom takes place, as seen in the bit of biologic behavior which has been mentioned as starting this inquiry, namely the death of the salmon after discharge of its sexual substances, this *defusion of instincts* becomes most notable and death takes place.

To quote Freud [9] on this point:

The Id, guided by the pleasure principle, that is, by the perception of "pain," guards itself against these (libido) tensions in various ways. It does so in the first place by complying as swiftly as possible with the demands of the non-desexualized libido; *i.e.*, by striving for the gratification of the directly sexual trends. But it does so further, and in a far more comprehensive fashion, in relation to one particular form of gratification which subsumes all component claims—that is, by discharge of the sexual substances, which are saturated conductors, so to speak, of the erotic tensions.

The ejection of sexual substances in the sexual act corresponds in a certain degree with the separation of soma and germ plasm. This accounts for the likeness between dying and the condition that follows complete sexual satisfaction, and the fact that death coincides with the act of copulation in some of the lower animals. These creatures die in the act of reproduction because, after Eros has been eliminated through the process of gratification, the Death Instinct has a free hand for accomplishing its purposes. Finally as we have seen, the Ego, by sublimating some of the libido for itself and its purposes, assists the Id in its work of mastering the tensions. There are certain people who behave in a quite peculiar fashion during the work of analysis. When one speaks hopefully to them or expresses satisfaction with the progress of the treatment, they show signs of discontent, and their condition invariably becomes worse. One begins by regarding this as defiance and as an attempt to prove their superiority to the physician, but later one comes to take a deeper and truer view. One becomes convinced, not only that such people cannot endure any praise or appreciation, but that they react inversely to the progress of the treatment. Every partial solution that ought to result, and in other people does result, in an improvement or a temporary suspension of symptoms produces in them for the time being an exacerbation of their illness; they get worse during the treatment instead of getting better. They exhibit the so-called negative therapeutic reaction. There is no doubt that there is something in these people that sets itself against their recovery and dreads its approach as though it were a danger. We are accustomed to say that the need for illness has got the upper hand in them over the desire for health. If we analyze this resistance in the usual way, then, even after we have subtracted from it the defiant attitude toward the physician and the fixation on the various kinds of advantage which the patient derives from the illness, the greater part of it is still left over, and this reveals itself as the most powerful of all obstacles to recovery, more powerful even than such familiar ones as narcissistic inaccessibility, the assumption of a negative attitude toward the physician or a clinging to the advantages of the illness. In the end we come to see that we are dealing with what may be called a "moral" factor, a sense of guilt, which is finding atonement in the illness and is refusing to give up the penalty of suffering. We are justified in regarding this rather disheartening explanation as conclusive. But as far as the patient is concerned, this sense of guilt is dumb; it does not tell him he is guilty; he does not feel guilty, he simply feels ill. This sense of guilt expresses itself only as a resistance to recovery, which it is extremely difficult to overcome. It is also particularly difficult to convince the patient that this motive lies behind his continuing to be ill; he holds fast to the more obvious explanation that treatment by analysis is not the right remedy for his case.

Now the issue that presents itself in the present suggestion is the direct corollary of all this, and in a sense the ambivalent. If one can hurt, that is, castrate the organ which is being used as the scapegoat, in whole or, preferably, usually in part, the punishment may be made to fit the crime, theoretically at least.

I am aware that the exact fitting into such a complementary relationship of a destructive process is not yet a matter of precise science. For many complex situations it is still a hypothetical issue, requiring further investigation.

We are faced, however, with some extremely interesting types of recovery from severe mental illnesses following acute somatic illness. Following an attack of typhoid fever, of influenza, of pneumonia, of accident, of severe operations, severe blood letting, severe purgation, even sometimes such minor events as tonsillectomy, appendectomy, thyroidectomy or teeth pulling, certain mental illnesses, often of long standing, have cleared up. The literature is vast and need not be summarized here. As yet, as stated, the relation of the disease process to the economics of libido displacement and instinctual fusion or defusion is not in exactly verbalizable form even if the principle be obvious.

For certain claimed results following colonic resection in schizophrenia, for example, one can follow the issues here outlined to advantage. Undoubtedly certain favorable results have taken place. They are not, in the opinion of the reasoning here sketched, the results of modifying "focal infection." The beneficial changes have resulted from a carrying out of the castration threat on a particular organ which has been made the specific medium for sadistic encystment of primary narcissistic libido, namely, the lower bowel. From the earliest days of the child's training the pleasure zone of the hostile, aggressive and sadistic components have been relegated to this area. The lower bowel and the motor apparatus are the chief primary organs for expression of sadism. The symbolism of the cities of the plains, Sodom and Gomorrah, as it was for the ancient Hebrews, still points to the chief abiding place of the unsublimated, homosexual, sadistic component of man's strivings. Here is, *au fond*, the avenue through which the " death wish " can find an outlet. In mutilating this organ (hemorrhoids for example) one punishes it; an " eye for an eye " retributory penance has been paid, and the instinctual conflict rearranged, sometimes to advantage.

In the case of certain chronic disabling somatic disorders, particularly in some of the atrophic arthritides, the motor organs, such as muscles, tendons, joints, are the chief agents for the carrying out of the sadistic impulses, and the defused and thus freed death impulse takes hold of and locks up the joints of such individuals in helpless bondage. Certain analyses of such organic processes, as yet fragmentary, show the same mechanisms operating as may be found in the neurotic criminal who must satisfy his need for punishment by getting in jail in order to assuage the sense of guilt which is derived from his Œdipus complex. The wheel chair of these arthritic types is the jail. Again here is no place to be dogmatic or for too widespread generalization, but with equal firmness it may be asserted that there is little doubt that certain atrophic arthritides become such as an outcome of the mental, dynamic factors briefly touched on.

One patient's history followed now for twenty years stands out from the point of view of this general discussion.

REPORT OF CASE

This patient, a member of an extensive family group in the United States with much eccentricity and genius in widely scattered branches and an apparently marked constitutional trend toward manic-depressive psychoses, had a definite small family history of this same type of reaction compromise. At least four in the immediate family had classic Kraepelin manic-depressive attacks and two others had somatic equivalents. Other more distinctly schizoid features were also present.

Cyclothymic reactions began at about the age of nineteen. The patient had just recovered, when seen in her late forties, from the last of three depressions which had been four years in duration. The " well " (?) period was characterized by much indigestion (much somatically, " treated " gastro-enterologically), incessant though fairly well regulated social activity, in which much sadistic-aggressive masked under a " great interest " in managing people was present. The aggression components were rendered less obnoxious by the frequent accompaniments of a mirthful, gay and even witty behavior when all was going well. A fairly persistent though often well hidden persecutory trend was apparent only to intimates. During this " well " period I was afforded time for exploration, but the transference always was of the negative type though carefully guarded. The early fixation factors were very obvious. The patient remained in this " well " state which Specht has described with great clearness in his contribution on paranoid states as part of the manic-depressive synthesis.

When it finally became definitely established that the object toward whom the patient's aggressive sadistic component were directed (the persecutor) would escape " justice," a depressed phase began to get into action. At first the sadism disengaged from its object chose, now one, now another external object, but to no avail. Then the aggression turned on its owner, and somatic disturbances were augmented, chiefly in the gastro-intestinal tract. They finally reached their acme and sequestered themselves in the gallbladder.

My surgical colleague called into consultation was of the ultra conservative type, and I was not as alert to the displacement dynamics of the holistic human animal as I now see it, and operation was decided against. The gallbladder attack subsided, and the patient went on to an eight-year period of deep mental depression.

As I now review the situation, I am hypothetically convinced that had we robbed (castrated) this person of the gallbladder, nature's effort at seeking a gratification of the death instinct through this channel would have been gratified, and a compromise through punishment and loss of an organ might have paid penance for the sense of guilt and averted this long period of depression.

This is not a statement that can be generalized beyond the special instance, especially in view of the fact that the whole series of mechanisms of sadistic displacement were quite well known to me. Further generalizations as to benefits to be derived from the operations should be carefully controlled, since it has been my experience to find that certain patients, most sorely involved in hopeless life conflicts, have utilized such operative procedures as a means for obtaining the unmodified death-wish and have died through such maneuvers rather than by the more conscious and obvious method of voluntary suicide.

In the case just mentioned, the gallbladder was the specially chosen organ for expression at the somatic level. In the language of a modern writer,[10] to quote rather than to paraphrase the hero's statement:

I had been chewing the bitter cud of remembrance, so bitter that it engendered the gall which, in the end jaundiced my vision of things that were past and things as they then existed; a gall that envenomed my emotions and tinctured my will, half paralyzing it.

And what was the product of all this? A venemous hatred, a futile revenge inspired by hate, a loathing of life as it had envisaged itself to

[10] Waller, M. E.: Windmill on the Dune. Boston: Little, Brown & Company, 1931, p. 147.

me, a disgust with the kind of (activity) that was demanded in the (social group).

A host of ancient and modern thoughts of similar implication might be gathered.

A brief sketch of an instinctively arrived at somatic castration may be added to round out this general thought.

In February, 1917, Dr. S. of B. referred to me a young woman, aged thirty, who was suffering from a psychosis then of several years' duration. It began in 1910 when she had to run away—psychically—from a marriage. She had a typical prenuptial flight into, first, a series of conversion symptoms, such as tachycardia, fainting spells, insomnia, dysmenorrhea and narcomania. She began to get physically run down and depressed, and finally had an acute confusional period in which she hallucinated, and for some months remained in a sanatorium in bed with the bed clothes pulled over her head (symbolic gestation). She then had delusional ideas of the loss of her insides. She was poisoned. She then carried a pillow under her arm, dealing with it as if it were a baby (symbolic delivery). While she was at the sanatorium a suicidal attempt was made. This confused period continued for several months more. She gradually became less restless and, not to unduly detail the history, by 1914, the whole affair became restricted to a negativistic, mute type of dependence, with delusional ideas of having killed her parents, both of whom were alive. She had been under the care of Dr. S of B. for three years in a sanatorium, where persistent gastrointestinal symptoms were treated, but little inroad on the delusional system had resulted.

Thus she came to me in the seventh year of a chronic psychotic process with manifest schizoid and definite depressed symptoms. She thus represented just that type of a psychosis concerning which Bleuler has frequently remarked relative to the diagnosis of schizophrenia and manic-depressive psychosis. The problem should not be put, has the patient schizophrenia or is he manic-depressive, but rather *how much schizoid and how much manic-depressive?* In short I was able to write to Dr. S. that this type of mixed psychosis, I believed, was more favorable for psychoanalytic therapy because of the mitigation of the more malignant process (schizophrenic) by the usually less malignant one (manic-depressive).

For six weeks the patient practically said nothing during her daily visits. I had to use an active technic and discuss her dress, her hat, her slightest finger, leg, neck and body movements, while outlining a general picture of the theory of psychoanalysis, interweaving these observations on her movements with the general principles. She then began to say something about her father and mother, why they were dead and why she was responsible for their death.

One of her recurring dreams had been that "her mother was dead." Her first reported dream after some weeks with me was of a "huge battleship without any guns" (castration of father and me).

Here the death of father and mother was not actual, but her remorse was " as if " she had killed them because of the hostile, sadistic, unconscious wish to castrate the father and take the place of the mother. The whole meaning of her symbolic birth fantasy during her stay in the hospital was thus introduced.

Little by little a working positive transference was established, and more and more history came out. The details do not concern this communication.

The final stand centered on the subject of a masturbatory displacement after about two years of treatment. For years she had had a small patch of a dry, scaly eruption to the left of the vagina which would itch, and she would at times scratch it almost to the point of bleeding. This she gradually came to realize was a masturbatory displacement, a remnant of an old overdetermined erotic phantasy. It represented a sort of sadistic, orgiastic gratification, in which the death of her mother and sister and the obtaining of her father and brother were fused in the one enterprise. We then had a very remarkable dream revelation of the whole situation, and following its analysis the patch became definitely infected, and the entire chain of superficial lymphatics in both groins became involved, which necessitated a surgical clearing out. Following this operation she went on to complete recovery and has now been well for over fourteen years.

In the language of the thought of this communication the patient finally sacrificed, by a castration mechanism, the chief remnant of her infantile Œdipus complex and was free. The body had attempted a previous death wish gratification by a suppurative appendix while she was in her suicidal state and before the complete development of her psychotic flight. Prompt operation had saved her life but not her reason. The analytic material at hand justifies this deduction. It would require thousands of words to demonstrate it adequately, and even then the report would be but a fragment.

IV

DUPUYTREN'S CONTRACTURE AND THE UNCONSCIOUS *

A PRELIMINARY STATEMENT OF A PROBLEM [1]

INTRODUCTION

For some time past the thought has been forcing itself into consciousness that I might like to say something about the human hand, something perhaps new, or novel, or different. But the longer I reflected and as more and more material, half-known, half-conjectural, came to the surface, the more prodigious seemed the affair. As through a glass darkly I loosely shuffled the scattered material dealing with the gradual ascending transcendence of the hands' activities throughout the primate series in its anatomic, physiologic, and psychologic advance. I knew where to start with the outlines of a monographic survey of the whole situation, but the longer I shuffled, the greater became my awareness of the futility of such an effort.

Then it seemed maybe one could limit the field and discuss just hands—the broad ones, the long ones, the fat ones, the thin ones; the leptosome hand, the pyknic hand, the thyroid hand, the pituitary hand, the eunuch hand; the artistic, the working, or whatever kind of hand, so intriguing to the pseudoscientific interests of the palmreader or other exploiter of human credulity.

Even here a monograph awaited the serious worker. So, throwing all such pretentious dreams to the winds, I would pick up a curious specimen and offer some possibly bizarre speculations concerning a chance finding turned up in the course of my daily work.

As many a stroll over the countryside has been temporarily halted by the sight of a unique botanical specimen which, on being brought home to the study table, has offered many hours of pleasant scrutiny and speculation, so, in the present instance, while delving intensively into the unconscious life of a sorely tried individual seeking relief from an agony of apprehension and of bodily distress, a unique type

* Reprinted by permission from Vol. III, 41st Series, *International Clinics*. Copyrighted, 1931, J. B. Lippincott Company, Philadelphia.

[1] This paper, in sketch, was prepared for a discussion at the Vidonian Club of Neuropsychiatrists, January, 1931.

of " hand specimen " here would claim some moments of reflection and fragmentary recording.

It is far from my intention to offer a monograph on Dupuytren's contracture. At the present time it is quite evident that the process that leads to the classic picture is far from being a unitary one. There are undoubtedly more than one series of factors involved in different cases, yet certain underlying possibilities offer an excellent opportunity for conjecture and research.

EARLY DESCRIPTIONS

It is not without a certain historic interest that the first physician who emerged from the scholastic morass of medievalism, so far as

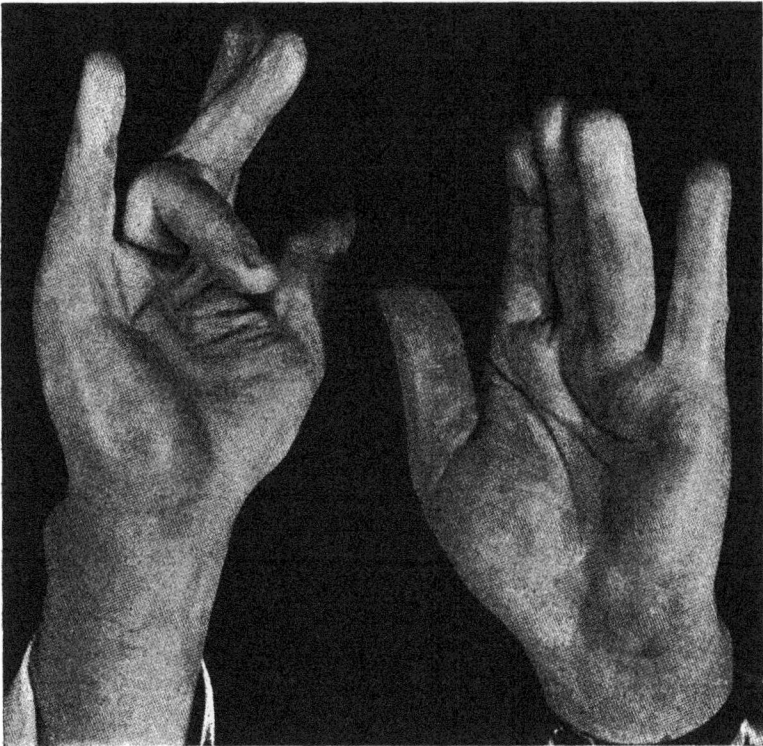

FIGURE 1

This is a picture of a patient of Dr. Bunnell's here reproduced, since my patient said it more truly represented his early condition, say at the age of thirty, than a score or more illustrations which I showed him. No one had ever taken a picture of his hands.

psychiatry was concerned—Felix Platter (1641)—is thought to have recorded the first instance of the kind of hand in question, and further, it may be stated that the present year is the one hundredth anniversary of the definite naming of the condition of which I would speak. In 1831, Baron Dupuytren clearly described and more accuratley outlined the essential integrity of the type of deformed hand which has since borne his name.

As with many new discoveries, controversy was rife. Dupuytren had to meet the orthodox giants of his day—Malgaigne and Velpeau—who tried to maintain that here was no new find. It was, they maintained, only an expression of a contraction of the tendons of the voluntary deep and superficial flexors. Dupuytren's masterly dissections of the palmar aponeurosis which showed the complete uninvolvement of the voluntary muscular attachments were sniffed at by the orthodox, until Langenbeck threw the weight of his authority on Dupuytren's side.

Dupuytren's careful dissections disposed of both deep and superficial tendon involvement. His early account is worth noting briefly.[2] In his " Lecons orales de Clinique Chirurgicale " it is stated (1831), "A man who for some time had been under the observation of M. Dupuytren, and was the subject of this deformity, died, and M. Dupuytren succeeded in gaining possession of the arm and hand. A careful drawing was made of the parts before the dissection. The whole of the skin was removed from the palm of the hand, as well as from the palmar surface of the fingers. The result was the complete disappearance from it of the folds into which it had been gathered. This opening out showed that its arrangement during the disease was communicated to it; but in what way or by what means was not evident. Continuing the dissection, the professor exposed the palmar aponeurosis, and was surprised to find it stretched, retracted, and shortened. From its inferior part were given off bands which passed to the sides of the affected finger. On making movements of extension in the affected fingers, M. Dupuytren observed that the aponeurosis underwent a kind of stretching and crackling. This threw light on the subject. It seemed clear that the aponeurosis was somehow connected with the deformity produced by the disease. The affected point remained to be discovered. The prolongations to the sides of the fingers were then divided; the contraction disappeared at once, and the fingers assumed their normal

[2] See Adams, W.: " Contractions of the Fingers," pp. 5–6. London, 1892.

condition of one-third flexion. The smallest force was now sufficient
to bring them into a state of complete extension. The tendons were
not implicated in any way, and their sheaths had not been opened.
All that had been done was the removal of the skin, and the division
of the bands of aponeurosis going to the bases of the phalanges.

"In order to remove all doubt and objections, M. Dupuytren dissected out the tendons. They retained their natural volume and
mobility, as well as the smoothness of their surfaces. Continuing the
examination, it was found that the articulations were in their natural
condition, the bones not enlarged, roughened, or presenting in any
way, either internally or externally, the smallest degree of change.
No alteration was observed in the apposition of the articular surfaces,
nor in their external ligaments; no anchylosis. Nor had the synovial
sheaths, or the cartilages, or the synovial membranes undergone the
slightest change. The conclusion naturally arrived at from these
conditions was that the starting point of the disease was the excessive tension of the palmar aponeurosis. As regards the cause of the
palmar lesion, it was considered to result from injury to the aponeurosis caused by the too violent, or too prolonged action of some hard
body held in the palm of the hand."

Since Dupuytren made this important contribution to our knowledge of this affection, in the year 1831, it has sometimes been spoken
of as Dupuytren's finger-contracture, a title as useful as it is also a
just compliment to the great surgeon, distinguishing it from all other
forms of finger-contracture.

Since 1831 there has been almost no question that the process
involving the palmar aponeurosis is a fibrosing, proliferative activity
affecting the connective-tissue elements with secondary contractures.
There are certain analogies to a fibrosarcomatous process which led
many dermatologists before and some few since to deal with the disorder among the dermatoses. Alibert and Jules Guerin were among
these. This general point of view has been entirely abandoned.

Practically all modern discussions of the problem speak of the
situation as *inscrutable from the standpoint of meaning.*

To present the present-day position a short description of Dupuytren's contracture is taken from the account written by Dr. Sterling
Bunnell for Dean Lewis' Loose Leaf Surgery, Vol. 3, p. 118, 1928.
This is chosen from the mass of literature as more to the point and
also for reasons to be noted later.

This condition is a progressive flexion contracture of one or more fingers, due to a fibrous hyperplasia and contracture of the palmar fascia and its digital prolongations. It is usually bilateral, one hand being affected earlier and to a greater extent than the other. Though it comes more frequently at the rheumatic age in men past middle life, it is occasionally seen in youth. Rarely it subsides spontaneously but as a rule is progressive and permanent. Heredity is a factor. One in four have some family history of it and Krogius reports its occurrence in fifteen descendants of one family. It is frequently associated with gout and osteoarthritis, and foci of infection and metabolic influences are possibly of more etiologic import than is trauma. Trauma no doubt aggravates the condition as tension and friction always increase fibrosis, but when we consider that it is no more frequent in manual than in non-manual workers and that the right hand is not affected much more than the left, it cannot be assumed that trauma is a prominent cause of the condition.

That some generalized condition is responsible is suggested by a case seen by the author in which bilateral Dupuytren's contracture and contracture of the fascial septal band between the corpus cavernosum and the corpus spongiosum of the penis occurred simultaneously.[3]

The contracture generally starts in the ring finger, then the little, middle, index and sometimes the thumb, in order of frequency. The contracting bands of palmar fascia stand out in the hand and radiate from the insertion of the *palmaris longus* tendon in the annular ligament. The bands can be followed down the fingers in lateral prolongations spanning the middle-finger joints to their attachment to the sides of the middle phalanx.

My patient, some of whose symptoms may be narrated later, had suffered since young boyhood with a gradually progressive Dupuytren's contracture in both hands for nearly forty years. It began in the right hand and then involved the other hand some years later, although it was never as intense in the left hand until recently.

He was about twelve to fourteen when he noted the difficulty first in the right hand and in the ring and little fingers of that hand—some time later, at least seventeen years, the left hand was involved. He is certain that his father had some of the same difficulty and also that his father's mother was likewise involved.

Nothing came out about the possible implication of the feet until

[3] Italics ours.

analyzing a dream, when it developed that one foot was also involved. He has no involvement of the penis.

Seventeen years previously a local surgeon operated on the right hand with much comfort, if not complete relief, for fifteen years, but in the past two to three years another operation was necessary and the left hand was also operated on to facilitate his game of golf.

Among the numerous contributions looking towards a deeper understanding of Dupuytren's contracture which might be utilized to throw light on not only the central psychologic conception here suggested but also illustrative of a principle that would aid in the understanding of the at times very striking heredity factor are papers by Krogius and Kajava which are of special significance. The former deals specifically with the problem of Dupuytren's contracture, the latter only with certain phyletic anatomic facts of the hand musculature.

Krogius, stimulated by the discussion of Kajava, believed that a more thorough central hypothesis was necessary than the traumatic (Dupuytren), gout, rheumatism, arteriosclerosis, tuberculosis, syphilis, alcoholic, central or peripheral nervous lesions, etc., all of which would herewith be discussed if a complete account were contemplated.

He was struck by the symmetrical involvement in both hands in most cases and also by the beginning history, either of fourth- and fifth-finger implication or in some isolated cases of the fifth finger alone starting the story, or being attacked alone. He quotes his twenty-two cases in the Helsingfor clinic, of which twelve were in both hands. In twelve the fourth or fifth or both fingers were involved. The others showed various modifications. In four of the families some hereditary history was obtainable. Involvement of four generations was found in one case.

Krogius states that Riedinger (1898) was among the first to show hereditary histories. He, however, would trace the somatic factor through sesamoid bone rests. Such are so infrequent as to render this conception very tenuous.

The Palmar Aponeurosis.—The developmental history of the construction of the palmar aponeurosis in man is still difficult to completely envisage. It is not the intention here to enter into the many uncertainties. It is not a simple connective-tissue sheet of unitary origin. For our purposes it is a compound of tendinous remnants from several phyletically more active muscles. The *Palmar longus* plays a large part in its construction. It may again be recalled that

Dupuytren's critics, Malgaigne and others, claimed the contractions were of the still active tendons, chiefly of the *palmaris longus*. Naturally in those days the principles attendant upon phylogenesis and modifications of older structures were only beginning to be grasped. The embryologic superficial sheet of the antibrachial flexors contains the anlage for the *palmaris longus* and the *flexores breves manus superficiales*. Thus the modified superficial short flexors also may contribute their aponeurotic quantum to the palmar aponeurosis. Only the *palmaris brevis* in this group of superficial flaxors of older mammals is occasionally found in man. Hence the fourth- and fifth-finger predominance.

In studies by Grafenberg the human embryo shows evidences of a *flexor digitorum manus brevis*. Although much of this muscle would seem to join the deep flexors—*flexor digitorum sublimis*—some of its superficial layers also enter into the palmar aponeurosis.

Whether other muscles of the superficial layer, important in lower forms of many mammals, enter into the construction of the palmar aponeurosis, it is not necessary here to go into greater detail. It is enough for the purposes of this paper to be certain that the aponeurosis consists chiefly of fibrous connective tissue of tendinous origin from phyletically appreciable muscular tissues which at one time were largely under cortical voluntary and cortical and striatal spinal reflex activities. (The whole problem of "reflex grasping" need not here be more than mentioned as of behavioristic significance. Critchley, Schilder, *et al.*)

Kajava (1917) in a study on the phylogenesis of the *palmaris brevis* and the *flexores manus breves* muscles in mammals showed that in many lower forms (Monotremata for example) whereas the *flexor brevis* muscles ran to four digits, in higher mammalian forms and up to lower primates the four and five fingers are alone so served, and that in the higher apes and in man these muscles are lacking. Only in anomalous rare cases can the *flexor brevis* be found running to the little finger. The *palmaris brevis* exists in higher forms chiefly as a superficial semi-muscular semi-aponeurotic flexor for the hypothenar eminence.

Grafenberg in his embryologic studies has pointed out that the *flexores breves manus superficiales* make up a fairly large and important muscular mass, which later is to be differentiated, during which some of the earlier mammalian utilizable muscle fibers fail as complete muscular structures but pass over into the construction of the fibrous bands of the palmar aponeurosis.

Thus Krogius came to the conception that phyletic hangovers, particularly of the short flexors, would account for the predominant involvements of the fifth and fourth fingers which is so evident and striking clinically.   Thus the heredity factor would receive support and explanation.

He further would think of the slow contractile process as a register of a tendinous regression of an undeveloped muscle anlage rather than a chronic-plastic inflammatory activity.

Our own more central dynamic conception could accept both processes as operative rather than one exclusively.

Krogius would summarize his study as being disposed to regard Dupuytren's contracture as due to developmental disturbances in the phyletic history of the superficial hand musculature (*Mm. flexores breves manus superficiales*).   Since the palmar aponeurosis must be considered in part a derivative of these in various mammals, and also occurring in the musculature of the human embryo, the newly developed tissues which fundamentally induce the contractures may be referred back to embryonic rests of the same muscular sheath.

The conception is not to be understood that true atavistic muscles have developed which in the disposed individual resulted in a tendinous modification of the same—but that the process is so conceived that the musculo-tendinous connective tissue incorporated in the aponeurosis develops in later life directly into the contractures.

As may be seen, Krogius goes only as far as *description*.   There is no dynamic conception anywhere that there is any " pull " on these *shadowy remnants of previous pullable structures*.   The forces that once brought about physiologic and useful activity through muscular and tendinous structuralized experience now are capable of causing pathologic useless crippling, as *unconscious " purpose " would reach back into the shadowy past and find only the remnants of what was once there.*

In a manner of speaking, then, it may be important to say that certain voluntary contractile *possibilities* as in the hands (and probably by homology in the feet) of lower mammals up to lower primates and even certain higher primates, are passing from conscious muscle-tendon contractile activity to " unconscious " aponeurotic contractile capacity.   In a sense such intermediary " conscious-unconscious " impulses will be more capable of producing results proportionate to two factors: The one somatic, and dependent upon the persistence of more musculo-tendinous tissue in those " heredity " families, and, the other, upon the nature of the development of the "grasping tendencies" of individual personality development. *This latter factor in its more detailed analysis is the newer, novel, or more completely developed conception which this paper would emphasize and offer supporting evidence from the psychoanalytic methodology.*

ABBREVIATED SYNOPSIS OF CASE HISTORY

It is not my intention here to enter into details of the general situation for which I was consulted. By reason of necessary restriction of an all-round presentation of the case history and the consequent picking out of the particular "hand-system-complex function" this, a preliminary study, must be viewed as a fragment only. In a rough sense, by analogy, I can offer but slight strains of a disjointed melody which flows within the body of a symphonic composition.

Believing as I do that practically all of the manifestations of the bodily functioning, physiologic or pathologic, must be viewed as a whole, then no single issue can be thoroughly understood without this "as a whole" conception. It is, therefore, an arbitrary procedure to pick out the Dupuytren's contracture should it be considered apart from the rest of the personality of the individual who harbors it. It will be seen, I hope, that *this particular pathologic manifestation is a consistent developmental product of the inner life of this individual.* It is a product of his "Id," *i.e.,* his deep unconscious, and its pathology, for him, and for *his case alone be it here emphasized,* becomes understandable. Even though I would thus avoid generalization and point out an individual pathology, the principle to be evolved, I believe, runs through most of the Dupuytren's contractures, even though other obvious factors, infectious arthropathies, syringomyelia, multiple sclerosis, spinal-cord or peripheral-nerve injury, etc., etc., accompany and may make possible the appearance of "Id" forces because of the loss of or hindrance to peripheral drainage factors. As I have previously discussed, *in extenso,* this coördinated emergent evolutionary picture of what has heretofore been set forth in parallelistic terms of somatic pathology and psychopathology, I shall refer this whole point to view to the interested by citation only.[4]

[4] With Dr. William A. White: "Principles Underlying the Classification of Diseases of the Nervous System," *Journal of the American Medical Association,* Vol. 66, p. 781, 1916; also see in Jelliffe and White: "Diseases of the Nervous System," Fifth Edition, Lea and Febiger, Philadelphia, 1929; Jelliffe, S. E.: "Paleopsychology; A Tentative Sketch of the Origin of Symbolic Function," *Psychoanalytic Review,* Vol. 10, p. 211, 1923; "Neuropathology and Bone

I first saw the patient in March, 1930. He was then fifty-two years of age. He came, through consultation, complaining chiefly of intolerable drawing sensations, chiefly in his arms. They were felt in the wrists, the elbows, the shoulders, also the back of the neck. The thighs and knees also had them. They were constant. There was tingling in the course of the nerves of the arms. The location of an, at times, " almost nauseating " tingling which was emphasized is shown here as complained of as of January, 1928. At times the finger-tips would tingle and have cotton-wool sensations, save when he lay down to sleep. His eyes bothered him also. He had drawing sensations there. He could not focus well.

The joints themselves were not stiff, he would explain, although he wanted constantly to " work them " as if to loosen them up or relieve him of the intolerable drawing-pulling feelings.

As far as could be learned, the " damned thing," as he expressed it, was of gradual evolution, was persistent, and was increasing. He had good days and bad days, good hours and bad hours. Certain attending factors here will receive further comment.

The eye symptoms apparently were the first, and it is possible although difficult to clearly pin down that these had an acute onset. This was in the summer of 1927 when he was salmon fishing in Canada. Here he had a " stomach upset "(?) with nausea. He awoke with acute retching, got up to urinate, was dizzy, things went around and around. He was forced to stay in bed, he thinks a few days. He is not sure but maybe he saw double at this time. At all events he felt " rotten " for a day or two. There was no headache recalled although he had had infrequent attacks of migraine with scotomata and nausea and headache—no ear ache.

Three or four days later he had a " rotten dizzy spell." He

Disease," *Transact. of the American Neurological Association,* p. 419, 1923; " Unconscious Dynamics and Human Behavior "; in Morton Prince Festschrift, page 231, Harcourt, Brace and Co., New York, 1925; an amplification of paper on " The Psyche and the Vegetative Nervous System with Special Reference to Some Endocrinopathies," *New York Medical Journal,* April 5, 1922; " Somatic Pathology and Psychopathology at the Encephalitis Crossroad," *Journal of Nervous and Mental Disease,* Vol. 61, p. 561, 1925; " Psychologic Components in Postencephalitic Oculogyric Crises " *Archives of Neurology and Psychiatry,* Vol. 21, p. 491, 1929; " Vigilance, the Motor Pattern and Inner Meaning in Some Schizophrenics' Behavior," *Psychoanalytic Review,* Vol. 17, p. 305, 1930; Groddeck, G.: " The Book of the It," Nervous and Mental Disease Monograph Series, No. 49; Groddeck, G.: " Our Unknown Selves," London, 1930.

thinks the tingling began about this time, possibly earlier, but it was hard to locate temporally because, from the old Dupuytren's contracture, he had always had a slight sense of pulling. Following the operations seventeen years ago (Dr. R——), and two years ago (Dr. P——), there were always peculiar sensory disturbances in the fingers.

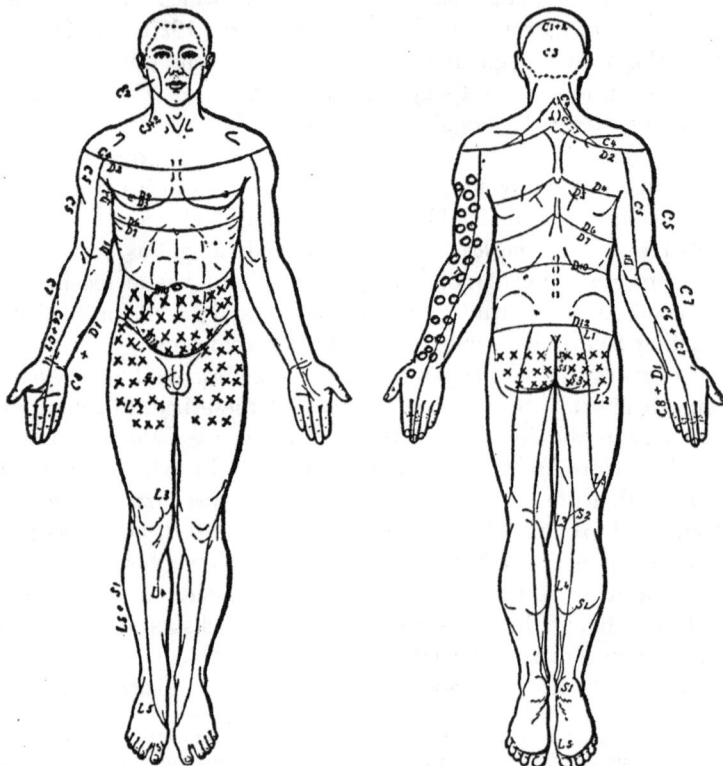

Figure 2

xx Location of almost nauseating tingling sensations.
oo Pulling tingling drawing in both arms but were more constant in areas indicated.   (March 30, 1930.)

His troubles continued.   He was an inveterate woodsman, hunter, and fisher.   He noted gradually advancing uncertainty in his wading the trout streams; the birds got away from his gun by reason of the blurred vision and focusing difficulties and slight initial motor checking. He grew more and more annoyed with petty hindrances to his enjoyment, and his apprehension and hypochondriac self-involvement grew on him. He anticipated impending dissolution, cerebral hemorrhage, heart failure (he had some extra systoles), blindness, paralysis, rheumatic disability, etc.

He consulted competent internists, surgeons, neurologists, X-ray specialists, etc., as early as March, 1928. One set of diagnoses at this time was, psychoneurosis, neurasthenia, benign thyroid tumor, and Dupuytren's contracture. Complete internist, neurologic, X-ray, metabolic and biochemic study revealed no marked variables from established " norms." The complete report is unnecessary in this discussion.

Since this time to when I saw him in 1930 other similar investigations were all " negative " so far as structural alterations were definable. He has a slight right corneal arcus-like cloudiness. That " reversible " to " irreversible " processes were going on is incontrovertible. The " why " of such a judgment affords the nucleus of this study.

In March, 1930, the patient, as stated, was fifty-two years of age. He was married twenty-eight years; was a successful professional man. There was a daughter of twenty-three, a son of twenty-one, and another daughter of sixteen. His father had died at seventy, kidney, when patient was twenty-two. His mother had died at the age of eighty-four. She was restless, nervous and twitching. His father had some Dupuytren's contracture as had his father's mother, he thought. There was a sister two years older than he and a younger brother. There are no outstanding familial variables, save the very neurotic mother.

Only a very brief summary of his childhood and adolescence can be offered. He was a happy, active boy much attached to his highly neurotic and restless mother, who, with the unmarried sister, became strong Christian Scientists. He was a possible bed-wetter. No other neurotic traits of childhood, save he used to sniff a great deal. He can recall the " habit " as early as seven or eight. He had many " colds " in the head from eight or nine to twelve or thirteen. He made good marks at a high-grade university, and took up his professional work, in which he has been progressively successful above the average. He always had a hankering for the woods—took frequent week-ends and short holidays, rationalizing his extra interest in motor activity, sports, living in the country, etc., as " healthful ";

" being nearer to family " ; and other well-accredited and widespread rational motives.

The unconscious material very early showed definite mother fixation factors. The father situation was not so quickly revealed, although it was soon apparent that the oral-sadistic pregenital phases of his libido situation were well invested.

The infantile oral-anal sadistic trends had developed chiefly along the motor pathway. Very briefly they were clearly separable into (1) an infantile cruelty phase and (2) the adult hunting, fishing, excessive motility, hustling, socialized, syntonic-get-together phases.

(1) *Infantile Phases.*—The sniffing and " colds in head " have already been alluded to. These belong in the nasal cathexis, displacements from behind-below to above-in front, *i.e.,* anal to nasal, as is so well known. Constipation was present. He also had some interesting sadistic plays when five, six or seven years old. He constructed a small guillotine with which he would chop off the heads of grasshoppers, etc. A little later he constructed a hangman's apparatus. He had a set of nine-pins with painted heads. There were the different types of men—merchant, minister, etc. ; these he would hang with considerable childish gusto.

There were a number of important variants of these cruelty plays, too involved to enter into in this short outline.

Oral fixation on the mother—appearing in not infrequent dreams of " twin objects " (breasts)—had led to an equally interesting character development. At his mother's knee he learned many poems, songs, etc. This fixation became a social asset in that he remembered literally thousands of poems, songs, stories, etc. This tenacity of memory—this holding—could be dilated upon to a marked degree. Whereas it never developed to the " miserly " stage as is frequently seen, nevertheless there were an innumerable series of small holdings, graspings, which are of significance in the whole hypothesis of " grasping " as related to the " hand " situation.

Much more might be written about the infantile " grasping " features of the pregenital erotic areas, but such would belong to a complete psychoanalytic presentation, which this paper is not.

As a genital phase of adolescence was reached, the conflict of masturbation arose. To develop this theme adequately would require many words.

That remnant of the unsolved Œdipus complex—as evidence the wish to castrate others (guillotine, hanging devices)—now threw up a hindrance to complete masturbatory development and gratification at the adult level. The sense of guilt was not particularly inhibiting in the Conscious when actual manustrupation began at eleven, but the evidence is strong that a marked defusion of instinctive object activity took place at this time. Detailed consideration of earlier homoerotic activities (seven, eight, nine years old) are omitted here, but the presence of such is noted as relevant to castration anxiety. Hence the displacement to and punishment of the left hand. The contractures began then in the left hand (twelve years). The " Id " would grasp with the right hand the Father Potency object with unconscious castration wish-intent, but a tyrannical Super-Ego bearing down forces the displacement of the libido, through denial, from right to left to the inner gratification of possession by grasping, thus subtly camouflaged. Thus the body is punished in true Pauline fashion. (The *lex talionis* principle " If thy right hand offend thee, cut it off," etc.) Details of the persistence of this all-powerful grasping tendency, through repressed masturbatory inner urge, cannot be entered into here. One dream bit of evidence alone is offered. Its complete analysis belongs to another phase of this presentation.

"*I am fishing in my favorite club stream, at the weir where the water is deep, just below the small falls. It is dark and the slightly foamy water is very attractive. The biggest fish are apt to be found in that place and I am anticipating getting some fine ones. Then in some manner I dry up the entire stream and I catch big trout in both my hands.*"

To those but slightly acquainted with dream mechanisms the strong grasping tendency shows itself here as a pregenital level combined with the masturbatory urge. Analysis of the dream, among other things, showed the pregenital urinary cathexis (water fall—biggest fish, in deep pool) and the later masturbatory object investment (grasping trout in both hands). The large amount of energy in the wish is adduced from the magic of drying up the pool. The relationship to the underlying Œdipus complex is also obvious.

As to the wished-for Father Potency factor which also shows up at a magic or mystic phantasy level, hence theoretically heavily invested, one or two bits of dream evidence may be noted.

In one dream: "*A half-horse half-man (Centaur) animal is anticipating coitus.*" (Other details omitted.)

This type of Centaur dream I have met with but rarely and thus far in my experience it has been found only in certain types of individuals who have in some more or less marked manner carried out some type of castration within their own bodies *(lex talionis)*. With me it has been found in three instances in patients with multiple sclerosis, with two who showed a progressive myopia, in one boy, twelve years of age, with diabetes, and in one epileptic girl. In two criminals of the neurotic criminal type (Alexander), *i.e.*, those who carry out criminal actions in order to be punished, I have also had such dreams. The theoretical implications of the animal dreams I have gone into in some detail in a previous paper.[5]

Leonardo da Vinci was the first great anatomist who really appreciated the muscle dynamics of standing. His drawings represent with faithful accuracy that the muscles utilized by a horse in rearing are the same as those used by man in rising from a stooping to an erect position and in keeping him erect.[6] I venture to assert that the " rearing Centaur " of the patient's dream life is an indication of a profound psychodynamic urge on the part of the patient to be greater than the father, *i.e.*, to possess in a surpassing degree the mounting capacity of the father, *i.e.*, have his infantile unconscious phantasied phallic power with the wished-for mother.

This particular patient never showed the interesting involvement of the penis found in other cases of Dupuytren's contracture which is here to be interpreted as related to this selfsame penis supremacy wish.

Since the earliest signs in this patient began at about the age of twelve, it is psychoanalytically interpretable that the masturbation displacement with its accompanying retribution reaction *(lex talionis)* afforded sufficient outlet for the repressed Œdipus situation. Just at what ages the fixations would tend to cluster in order to bring about the unconscious actual penis castration (by bending) details of the available histories do not permit of any adequate analysis. Should the opportunity offer, further inquiry concerning these unique case histories may be carried out.

One other feature of the Centaur position, or more properly speaking, the animal-coitus position, as an index of infantile theories of coitus, and also related to incompletely sublimated anal-sadistic phantasies, another dream may throw light upon this investment as

---

[5] With Brink, L.: " Rôle of Animals in the Unconscious." *Psychoanalytic Review*, Vol. 4, p. 250, 1917.
[6] *Cf.* Murrich: " Leonardo da Vinci, the Anatomist," 1930.

bearing upon the "nauseating tickling" sensations of which he complained. In this dream, "*Coitus was being attempted from behind, but great care was being exercised* [and this was emphasized by the dreamer in telling it] *not to penetrate the anus.*" This is but part of the dream. Bearing on this infantile animal position material also were dreams of unmistakable character. "*Two dogs in such position but kissing each other in unmistakable human character, with almost clear glimpses of smacking lips.*"

The parts of the body which would be brought in skin apposition—*tactile skin erotism*—a large factor in this contractile palmar aponeurosis—are shown in the accompanying charts. (Fig. 2, page 46.) It is of psychologic import to note that in these "nauseating sensations" the patient is both subject and object. That the vulgar jargon should have an adequate phraseology for this retributive activity is not without considerable significance.

It would lead to too great piling up of detail were all of the situations relative to great impatience, at times childish, irritable behavior when thwarted, even in minor games of backgammon, bridge, etc.; ever-present persistent and markedly titanic desires to anticipate, to hurry, to get hold of things before it were possible, or lest he be thwarted. Jink's, and other gestures, oaths, rituals, superstitious observances galore exemplify the infantile stages of libido cathexes which have had a partial liberation through the grasping, holding activities through the hands but by reason of inadequacy of performance at really creative levels have flowed into the vegetative effectors and old connective-tissue metamorphic products of what were in lower animals tendinous capacities for such holding, grasping, reflex activities.

V.

THE PSYCHE AND THE VEGETATIVE NERVOUS SYSTEM *

WITH SPECIAL REFERENCES TO SOME ENDOCRINOPATHIES

To state the fact that man is a social animal smacks of the obvious. One so often meets with the inference, however, that he is a mere chemical test tube that it seems necessary to emphasize the concept of his preëminent social function. The hypothesis which works best, that is, that which explains the most phenomena, regards him as an evolutionary product with an enormous ancestry. That ancestry began with cosmic physical and chemical forces. They still remain determinants for aftercoming reactions. When life first insinuated itself into dead matter ; when crystalline laws were surpassed, because they were too rigid to allow for newer adaptations, a type of super-chemistry arose, the behavior of which science has symbolized under the term *vital* and which became condensed in structure. Vital structures in their turn threatened to limit the development of life's accumulations. The inexorable fact of duration, that " piling up of the past upon the past," with its inevitable necessity for hanging on to the entire past, forced a supervitalism which finally in man was met by the masterly invention of the symbol, by which this mighty Atlas of the past might be compressed, in tablet form as it were, to be used in the social machinery. Its most intelligible form is language, although that is not its only product.

Then when we speak of the psyche we here mean that function of man which operates by means of and through symbols, and psychical mechanisms are chiefly symbolic mechanisms. Their study is the study of symbology with its enormous phyletic past which is just being unraveled. By many who are mostly dealing with classroom

* Reprinted by permission from the *New York Medical Journal* for April 5, 1922.

Abstract of a Clinical Lecture, delivered at the Post-Graduate Hospital Medical School, Sessions of 1911–12. (The main outlines of this paper were given in 1912 in a lecture at the Post-Graduate Hospital. It was revised and presented in abstract at the American Neurological Association in 1914. For reasons of discretion, some of the situations being recognizable at the time, publication has been deferred.)

problems, this study is more often called psychology. The average classroom psychology, however, only commences to fringe on the actualities of life. The psychology that is of any service is that which has this enormously rich past, of which the previously emphasized evolutionary hypothesis takes cognizance. It is the psychology which is tucked away, condensed, compacted in the symbol. It is best termed the psychology of the unconscious, or as Bleuler (1) has termed it, deep psychology. Only by such a concept can we get into sympathetic touch with the past.

The unconscious contains all of the chemistry, the vitalism, and the symbolism. It has everything from the beginning. The psychology of the conscious is but a momentary flash of what the hundred million years of life have concealed in the living human being. It expresses only the numerator of the fraction which represents life. The immensely more important part of life, which is hidden, is the denominator, *i.e.*, as the numerator one second is to the denominator, one hundred million years, so is our conscious knowledge of what is going on to that which really makes it happen (the Unconscious).

Bergson, in his inimitable way, says: " It is with our entire past that we desire, will and act. Our past then is made manifest to us in the form of impulse, it is felt in the form of tendency, whereas only a small part of it is known as idea." It is, then, as readily may be seen, a long jump from the idea, the symbol, back to the beginning of things in man, the vegetative nervous system.

From the evolutionary attitude the vegetative nervous system looks after the chemisms of the human body, hence its function is related to the earliest part of the past in the unconscious denominator. The phyletically oldest part of the vegetative nervous system, and that part which still maintains the loosest of structural relationships, is the endocrinous gland system. Some of these glands have manifest morphological resemblances to nervous structures, such as the pineal, the hypophysis, and parasympathetic ganglia, while, others, such as the prostate, pancreas, and thymus, have no obvious neurological affiliations. A distinctly advancing series may be made out in which the resemblances increase. Such a series, from the least to its most obvious nervous similarities, would be prostate, testicles, ovary, thymus, thyroid, parathyroid, pancreas, choroid plexus, suprarenals, neuroglia, sympathetic paraganglia, pineal, and hypophysis.

It has been assumed by many physiologists that each of these structures elaborates some specific substance to which the name hormone (energy carrier) has been applied by English physiologists. Although only one of these hormones has thus far (1911) been definitely isolated, epinephrine (adrenaline), yet it seems fairly well demonstrated that substances specific in some sense at least exist within each of the structures mentioned. Kendall's thyroxin is possibly another.

It is quite probable that intracellular chemism in simple cellular organisms is largely a physical and chemical affair. The colloidal state of the protoplasm permits this. But with succeeding complexities channelings became essential; these, foreshadowed in the fibro-vascular bundles of the plant, finally slowly progressed into the vascular, muscular, neuromuscular, and nervous structures of the adult vertebrate.

The chief hormones in these higher animals are now carried through the body by means of the blood current, and there occurs an amazingly complex interplay between the vascularly brought hormone supply and the individual need, in which the receptor end of the nervous arc touches the need reality, and the effectors end makes the appropriate and adequate response in trophic, secretory or motor action.

Carbon dioxide is the original and phyletically the oldest of the hormones; Parhormones, Gley prefers to call them. The phylogenesis of its successors has not yet been traced. Physiology is looking for a Mendelieff to trace out the hormone evolutionary products. A better knowledge of the chemical evolution of our present hormones is still lacking. I can refer you to no studies on the subject, as I have never seen it broached, but I feel certain that such must exist, but these need not detain us. Nevertheless, while dealing with carbon dioxide, let us stop a moment here and point out a relationship between it and respiration and the further function which man has developed as an accessory to his carbon dioxide hormone need, namely, aspiration, which is chiefly discussed as human speech.

The lung function, hormonely speaking, is closely related to the psychical function of social integration through symbolic language. I shall hope to raise several concepts for your consideration relative to the psyche and to the vegetative nervous system, which are, I believe, very pertinent in human pathology. For just as man cannot live simply to eat, so the man who utilizes his lungs only to breathe will surely die. He must do something more with them. They form a part of the mechanisms for his creative energy, and through the expression of ideas he really lives. In terms of the parable of the talents, if he simply wraps up his respiratory gift in a napkin and does not put it out to usury, *i.e.*, to create and exchange ideas with his fellow man, he will be in the position of the one who " hath not and shall have taken away from him even that which he hath." I beg of you not to get ultrascientific—criticism usually being thought of as science by many—and remind me that deaf mutes can live.

When I hazard the expression of my conviction, concerning which I may devote an entire lecture, that the problem of the conquest of the chief enemy of the respiratory organs, the tubercle bacillus, is taking place through a better and better distribution of respiratory psychical energy—libido—I trust you will take it as something to think about and study in your individual cases along lines which it is the general purpose of this lecture to outline. If I were able to trace for you, step by step, the psychology of the unconscious so far as respiratory needs were concerned, I think we could see the pathology of tuberculosis, and many respiratory affections with an enlarged vision. The old truths are still true, but inadequate. I think that I shall be able to do this for certain asthmas for we know enough of these cases to be able to show some of the unconscious mechanisms which probably interfere with harmonious suprarenal activity, and thus bring on the asthmatic spasms.

Just here I border on an extremely important topic. I have approached it through a respiratory pathway, but it could have been approached by a number of different avenues. Shall we say, as I have preferred to phrase it, that the unconscious mental mechanisms induced a modification of the suprarenal glands or other hormone producing bodies, which in their turn so changed the vegetative nervous system control of the respiratory organs—unstriped musculature, as to induce an asthmatic attack, or shall it be phrased, as it most frequently is, that a disorder of the suprarenal gland alone or with other related endocrinous glands has brought about the altered action of the vegetative nervous system, and thus caused the asthmatic attacks, leaving the psychical situation out entirely.

Here it is that I wish to emphasize the importance of the title to this lecture. In the first place, there is not the slightest doubt that there are asthmatic attacks in which neither the psychical system nor the hormone systems are involved. Such attacks are due to direct involvement of the sensorimotor structures themselves, from tumors, caseous nodules, or syphilitic processes within the posterior mediastinum pressing upon the main nerve trunks. Then again there are other endocrinous neurological disturbances, asthma being only one in which the involvement is primarily of endocrinous origin. These are due to acute inflammations or other direct somatic implication of an endocrinous gland. But, and here is the chief point in our discussion, there are also certain other affections of the vegetative nervous system which are preëminently or even solely psychogenic in their origin. Surgery or pharmacotherapy is essential for the first group and other therapies are illusory. Psychotherapy is hocus pocus for the second group and opotherapy or X-ray therapy is indicated, while for the last group psychotherapy is alone rational and other therapies are usually buncombe.

To which group, or rather to what preponderance of action, a given disturbance belongs can be determined only after a most painstaking neurological analysis, with special methods devised to determine the specific vegetative nervous system anomalies, as well as a thorough acquaintance with the conscious and unconscious life of the patient. It is of no avail to speak of neurasthenia, or psychasthenia, or hysteria, or dementia praecox, or autointoxication; these are not terms which explain anything. In this connection it may be said that these expressions are too frequently the refuge of ignorance, which largely permit the practitioners to do what they find easiest to do, rather than what should be done for the patient. Above all, do not be thrown off the track by the cheap trick of the superficial dogmatist who pooh poohs that which makes man what he is, the psychical as well as the metaphysical subtleties.

In a previous lecture we discussed certain methods of investigating the vegetative nervous system which have come into use in the past five or six years, and which promise to aid us greatly in sizing up a large group of patients who have been much neglected because of the inconstancy and bizarreness of their symptoms.

Few will be in doubt concerning a diagnosis of cretinism or myxedema, of exophthalmic goiter, Addison's disease, diabetes, acromegaly, dwarfism, achondroplasia, Raynaud's disease, scleroderma, or psoriasis. Yet it must be emphasized that for every single evident and well marked vegetative disturbance (2) there are one hundred atypical, irregular, incomplete or mixed cases.

I am inclined to believe that fully 50 per cent of the cases which now are frequently looked upon as abortive or mild cases of hypothyroidism or hyperthyroidism, ten years ago were diagnosed by the selfsame physicians as neurasthenia. I have done so myself in many instances, and with each periodical revision of my histories, following out the later histories, I find many important things which were entirely overlooked. Ten or twenty years in the future there will be a different way of grouping the accumulated facts, each new generalization, symbolized by a diagnosis, helping " more of the patients- more of the time " than the preceding ones.

Case History

Case.—A woman, thirty-five years of age, of Scandinavian parentage. She had been married about fourteen years and had one child, a girl four years of age. Her husband had a good retail business, was moderately prosperous, a hard worker, and left her much to herself. About five years ago she had her first upset, with a mild exophthalmic goiter. This quieted down but during the whole time she was nervous, easily fatigued, and from the time she came for treatment, a period of three or four months, was a typical vagotonic neurotic. She had a slight struma, somewhat larger on the right side, which became worse following an attack of tonsillitis, to which disorder she stated she had not been subject.

She was slightly agitated, had a very fine tremor, her face was slightly flushed, and there were reddish patches on the skin. The eyes were not markedly protruding, the palpebral fissures were slightly unequal, the left somewhat larger than the right, the pupils were unequal, and her eyes glistened. As she looked down the eyelids followed slowly. There was no tachycardia. She said she had some respiratory hunger and felt oppressed at times. There was a sense of globus hystericus and examination showed the presence of some visceroptosis. She had lost fifteen or twenty pounds in weight and had attacks of looseness of the bowels without diarrhea. Her blood pressure was fairly high. She was vivacious in her manner, lively, and inclined to laugh and be happy. She said she slept poorly and dreamed little. Internists had told her she was suffering from autointoxication. Eosinophilia was 5 per cent, but gastrointestinal therapy had been inefficacious. Rest in bed had not been of particular service.

Attention might be directed to the fact that she had an increased suprarenal reaction, a mild hyperadrenalemia, also a mild hyperthyroidism. If statistics were being collected from the adrenal point of view, she would be the former; if from the thyroid, the latter. If one had just been reading Cannon's work on the reciprocal relation between the adrenals and the thyroid, it might be assumed that these glands were overfunctioning. From the knowledge that the patient had had tonsillitis which was followed by an exacerbation of her symptoms, one might assume the presence of an infectious thyroiditis of a mild grade. Any and all of these points of view would be perfectly valid. At all events, her tonsils should be cleared up and possibly X-ray applications might help a possible infection. The patient might be given a rest cure or a surgical operation but

I hazard the opinion that if one went no further the woman would not be helped very materially. She would probably move into another hospital or go to another doctor.

Let us turn, however, to her psychical condition and see what a sorry mess she is in and learn something about an essential element in the case. If you neglect this you really know nothing about her. On a previous occasion I referred to the occurrence of an acute hyperthyroid state directly following a sudden money loss and I venture the suggestion that conscious and unconscious money conflicts are often highly important emotional factors lying behind a hyperthyroidism.

This patient was married, not for love, but, as she expressed it, her family thought it was a good match and she was almost shoved into it. She went through with it, however. The marriage was so-so, but as she was excitable and her husband precipitate and always too busy to be with her much, she was mostly unsatisfied. "He did not marry her for that," he would say. She managed to get along, however, presenting only mild anxiety neurosis symptoms for which she was "bromided" for about ten years by numerous physicians, who called her hysterical. She remained sterile throughout this period, at no time taking any precautions or preventives. Much could be said about her creative wishes—unconscious—all this time. Of course there were curettages. The only really interesting thing was that for a time she menstruated every fourteen days. This I correlate, with apologies to my gynecological confrères, with the unconscious wish for a child.

She then had a little love affair with one of her admirers and that month became pregnant. She had had intercourse with her semipotent husband and her lover the same week, and it was when she commenced to worry as to whose child it was, whom it would look like when it grew up, what her husband would think, whether he would throw her out, and a host of other extremely disturbing doubts and inquiries, that the first attack of hyperthyroidism (and tonsillitis) came on. She was in an extremely agitated state for some time. Whether it was the thyroid that produced the agitation or the agitation that produced the hyperthyroid activity, I leave for you to decide. She was perturbed for some time during the pregnancy. Luckily all of the triangle were blue eyed and light haired and not being disturbed by any knowledge of Mendelian recessive factors, she finally came to a moderate state of adjustment. The hyperthyroidism slowly disappeared and she "carried on." For a time, during the nursing, she was better. Her husband was much more attentive and although he was still far from being potent she managed to get along presenting only some anxiety neurosis symptoms. Of late, however, the husband had been very busy and, as he had to get up very early in the morning, he had to go to bed early in the afternoon or evening. Little by little he left her more and more alone. He was exhausted from his day's work and at times would go months without intercourse, and when he did attempt it, it was finished in a second. She either masturbated or developed anxiety symptoms and phantasies.

Some years later we faced a new and severe flareup. Just what determined this flareup, I do not think the ordinary methods of inquiry would give us any genetic clue, not even the Goetsch test or her basal metabolism, so let us turn to the dream life during the period of the beginning of this recurrent attack and see what it may show. The reason for this type of inquiry I have tried to point out at various periods but let me repeat here the general thesis that is followed.

The individual as a whole is the subject of our inquiry at this particular time; we are not interested in any of its parts, save indirectly. As a whole, the human being functions in his *wish capacity;* he is constantly forming plans to carry out desires and cravings. In a specific way we may state that of these desires and cravings there are two chief modes of expression. They follow two broad roads, as it were, which run parallel toward a goal which, for lack of a better term, let us call happiness. I might change the metaphor and say that this stream of wishes could be compared to a twisted strand of rope made up of innumerable intertwined smaller strands in which two large groups of strands could be distinguished. These roads, these strands, following the German poet Schiller's example, we roughly call hunger and love. They constitute the great wish forces of life. Self-preservation and race propagation are their ancestral and present day patterns. Do we eat to live, or do we live to eat? An answer to this question tells us that whereas life's energy flows more strongly now through one, now through the other, yet if one could put a pressure gauge upon these two forces, I believe the highest pressure would be found on the race propagation side, and the old dictum that self-preservation is the first law of Nature would be found to be false. The phylum, the race, is more important than the individual. In the swing of Nature's pendulum which oscillates alternately but never just equally, for Nature does not relish being caught on a dead center, the push is greater on the race propagation side. The fly wheel of the race propagation side is loaded. Creative evolution is thus made possible and the game goes on. It has come from protozoon to man, a lively contest of new models for anywhere from one hundred to a thousand million years. During all this slow ascent organic memory has been laying away useful bits of biological structure, building them finally into a fabric which we call man. These old bits of structuralized function, for this is what the organs of the body can advantageously be conceived of as being, contain much that is not available to conscious control. They function automatically, yet are not out of actual contact with the rest of the body.

The body as a whole is an organization of all of these, a synthesis made possible by the nervous system. Not at the receptor surfaces, not in the spinal cord, not in the midbrain, not in the motor or sensory cortical projection fields, but only finally in the frontal cortex is this ultimate synthesis made effective. Here intuition or instinct meets with intelligence. Control of the bodily movements to satisfy its cravings has an arbiter. This control factor, however, has been building itself up just as long as any organization was found to be an advantageous scheme of things. When there were no conflicts, intuitive action went straight to its goal and satisfaction was implicit. When obstacles arose, however, then a new scheme of things arose. We called it consciousness. It was a byproduct of faulty intuitive action. It was only needed because intuition became clouded. The unconscious, for such can be named the vast series of intuitive, instinctive syntheses, tended to be blocked by as yet illy assimilated conscious contacts. Man's intelligence and his instinctive reactions were in conflict, and his vaunted intelligence was wrong. When we say that conscience doth make cowards of us all, are we not only saying that the unconscious is wiser really than our intelligence?

Beyond Good and Evil is the title of a study by Nietzsche. He has seen that force, neither good nor evil, is present within our unconscious. How shall we utilize that force? For good or for evil? That determines health or illness! Then our unconscious is very badly maligned. Yes, it is. It is the source of both good and evil, yet it is neither.

What then is good, or evil? Everyone has asked the question. So long as mankind dealt with conscious psychology anybody could make his own definitions, and everybody did. What is one man's meat is another's poison, and we have every possible brand of good and evil, according to climate, to race, to custom, and to fashion. From this point of view my doxy is orthodoxy and your doxy is heterodoxy. Everybody who thinks differently from me will be damned. So has mankind come up, getting freer and freer from certain dogma, and yet chaining himself tighter and tighter to other dogma.

In the unconscious, however, will be found truth in simple form. Here we can see what we are after without all the currents and countercurrents of camouflage and hypocrisy. The dream is the royal road to the unconscious. Such is Freud's well known and well tried out suggestion. We shall, therefore, look to the dream.

The first day I saw the patient I obtained a full history of her family, her father, mother, brothers and sisters. Her mother had always kept an eye on her. As to her dreams she told me she rarely dreamed. A great many people say the same but everybody dreams just as everybody breathes, secretes bile or urine but not all people *remember* their dreams. As to nightmares, she said she had had one recently. It was as follows:

She was going to a party. She had a lovely time. She was glad to see a stranger. (She awoke with palpitation.)

I did not attempt analysis of this nightmare and shall not now, only remarking that the word " party " had a double significance. She saw a stranger and she woke up. Whether the wish was to have a party with a stranger and that gave her nightmare—for it will be recalled how a similar " party " gave her a " baby "—I shall leave for the moment and go to the next dream. For we must be interested in the specific rather than the general problem.

At the next visit she recalled with some difficulty the rambling dream she had had the night before. She dreamed as follows:

I met a man on an elevated station. It was at ——— Street, where there was a shuttle train [going backward and forward]. *He did not recognize me. Then there was a lady there whom he seemed to know. I was with someone then, and as I watched them I said to this someone, a woman, " Oh, if Mrs. P.* [the wife of the man] *should know this." I decided it was the best policy to say nothing about it.* (She had anxiety and some palpitation when she awoke.)

This dream was also only cautiously dealt with. Mrs. P., it came out, was a woman who kept a " fashionable boardinghouse."

NOTES ON THE DREAM

Q. *"Mr. P.?"* A. " Oh, he was her husband. He spoke several languages. He had kept a hotel. He ran around with many women. His hotel was foreclosed. She was a hard working woman. She had had some business with Mrs. X.'s [the patient's] husband. Her husband, Mr. X., was greatly worried about business. He might be foreclosed. He was thinking of moving or changing his business somewhat, had thought of supplying delicatessen to hotels."

Q. *" What comes to your mind about shuttle?"* A. " He got out at ——— Street. I was going to take the *downtown* train."

Q. *"The woman Mr. P. seemed to know?"* A. "Oh, she seemed to be someone I knew. A fast woman. She was a fly person. She laughed and giggled. She was short and stout." [Patient was tall and thin—disguise of censor—fair—patient was fair.]

Q. *"What comes to your mind?"* A. "I've lots of friends, I know lots of people. I know no friends like her. Mrs. d. V., she's a little suspicious. But I'm broadminded, I don't believe in being narrowminded. Of course, people like that, they must live—what sort of a life? How much nicer and how much worse it must be. She is beautiful [patient was a handsome blonde]. People have different ways of living, after all. Terrible, in a way, but then they can love one another. A mistress, sometimes may be possible. Companions, they can get away from each other when they get on each other's nerves. Still a married woman is the best. It is safer."

This then leads to a long discussion as to her young womanhood and her girl friends, and the "fellows" that called. She liked life and wanted a good time, but with X., he was all for business. He never liked to be gay. He was tired all the time. She wanted to go out, play cards, dance, see the shows. But my mother, she had her heart set on my marrying a steady fellow. I respected him highly. He was always very serious. He never flirted at all. He is very kind, but is not my real mate. At first everything was terribly painful (dyspareunia). After a few months it was all right, but he never seemed to care much for "that." "Had not married me for that." Practically always unsatisfied.

I have presented the chief features in the dream, and have given some of the free associations of the dream. I think as you revise this material it will be quite clear that the patient was seriously disturbed over the temptation of being some man's mistress. She was resisting it, as the free associations tended to show—"A married woman is safer," etc. I did not disturb the patient too unduly, and I did not attempt to bring into consciousness whose mistress she wanted to be, but let her tell all about her troubles with her mother, about her husband and the hard work she had to go through on account of the baby, the difficulty with maids, with the cook, her husband's irritability, etc.

Then for a few days she had no dreams. Then a few about the child. In one dream, *her girl had peculiar white and green stools which worried her.* These were also left only partly analyzed. It is of very little service in a beginning analysis to try to show a woman that her child, especially a girl child, may be a nuisance to her, from certain aspects of her personality. Such truths can only be discussed when the patient knows more about the selfishness of her Id and its conflict with her better self, *i.e.,* her love for her child.

Then she had a dream of *having triplets, two blondes and one with black hair and brown eyes.* This brought out a great deal about her fears about whether the child she had had was her husband's child or the lover's child. If her lover had brown eyes and black hair what would have happened? There was much material, but I waited feeling certain that I would soon find the man with the brown eyes and the black hair. I did not get anywhere for two weeks.

One of the dreams in the interim contained material which dealt with a doctor who curetted her and who had been very friendly. Her transference to him was very strong and the dream discussed whether I should be entitled to as close a place in her confidence as Dr. Z. Two or three neurologists she had consulted also appeared in the dreams.

In about six weeks after I had begun to see her she presented the specific situation. She dreamed: *There were two gray automobiles standing in ——— Street* [the street where she lived], *between ——— and ———* [parallel streets, *i.e., parallel wishes*]. *One was all adorned with draperies, with bright colors on the body. There were red bandannas in it. " I don't like this car. Like a fortune teller's wagon." Out of each one came a Mr. L. with a woman. She was a fast woman. There was another woman and another man I knew. Both go to Mr. L.'s house. Then I say if Mrs. L. were alive what would she say?* Then in another dream the same night: *I visited Mrs. L. She was alive and the place was very upset. " It looks as if you were going to move," and she picks up some artificial hair, puts it on her head. It was black in color, and she said, " Is it not awful the way my husband abuses me?"*

I felt justified in bringing the issue up on this situation, and from the dream associations it soon developed that Mr. L. was the dark haired, brown eyed man who was trying to persuade her to be his mistress. He was a widower, a lawyer, wealthy(?). There was some doubts about his generosity, as a previous dream about *rings and jewelry* had partially revealed; he was rather stingy with his money, and, also possibly as a lawyer, he would get out of the *divorce possibility with her husband,* and leave her stranded after all.

It would be nice to exchange her situation with an automobile situation (wealth and comfort) but (red bandannas) was he only a *slick fortune teller,* after all, and where would she land in the interchange when she went to Mr. L.'s house as mistress (urged) or as wife of wealthy man (promised)?

Of course, for ordinary mortals without such temptations (for remember she had a husband who neglected her) there is little need to be agitated and disturbed, but for her, as she used to go to the lawyer's office to discuss the possibilities of divorce, and he would make passionate love to her "on his very ample sofa," it does not take a wizard (fortune teller, myself) to see her dilemma.

Now, I could elaborate this complicated story into a three volume novel, and novelists deal with just such realistic (human) material, and we sit up into the small hours of the mornings reading them. Why? Because as novelists, they put it all into intelligible terms, while we, as scientists, deal with the impulses that need all these terms to render them intelligible to mankind. As a scientist, I bring before you only the bare framework of the forces which are pulling this woman. Her cravings and her fears, money, comfort, automobiles, sexual satisfaction on the one hand; a secure home, her daughter, her marriage security, meaning social support, on the other.

Why should we consider the hyperthyroid activities as a mediating mechanism? I do not know. If I did know, possibly I would know as much as God knows, and with all my pretensions to knowledge, I have not yet gone so far as to approach the Omnipotent. All we can say is that here is a definite series of wish components on the one hand, and an equally definite series of bodily reactions on the other. If Pavloff's dogs show gastric juice reactions to conditioned stimuli, and Cannon's cats show somatic reactions to other types of stimuli, can we not say that the "prostitution-mistress-money-comfort" stimuli have something to do with the hyperthyroid physical reactions? I seriously ask you to consider the possibilities, yes, the probabilities of this connection. It is a specific stage of the parental complex.

And here we must leave it, but before I leave it I can not refrain from alluding to an important reflection. The situation, on the outside, and partly from the inside, is very widespread. Many human beings are caught in just this kind of a dilemma, yet hyperthyroid reactions do not develop in all. I can only say: So be it. I agree with you absolutely. There must be a definite chain of events which lead to a definite outcome. Is this hyperthyroidism alone conditioned by the factors which I have all too hurriedly sketched? I do not think so. There are constitutional factors which are a part of the structure. These are to be resolved as well, but in the meantime while we are busy with the biochemical and hereditary part, we are faced with the present, real situation. The patient wants, and yet does not want, to run away with the dark haired, brown eyed man; sacrifice the husband and the daughter; and get even with the mother who had always bossed her, and who had thrust this worthy husband upon her. Can she stand it? She can not! Her somatic disease is her conscience, God's law, her sacrifice.

We as physicians must first straighten out her ethical conflict. Removing her thyroid does not do this, even if we admit that she has gotten her body into such a mess that she would rather die than renounce the *wish*. For this happens and only surgery may prevent the unconsciously arrived at somatic suicide. What happens afterward, even if the thyroid be removed?

REFERENCES

1. BLEULER: *Jahrbuch für Psychanalyse,* ii.
2. JELLIFFE and WHITE: Disorders of the Nervous System, Vegetative Levels. Lea & Febiger, Philadelphia, 1915; third edition, 1919.

VI.

THE BODILY ORGANS AND PSYCHOPATHOLOGY *

I am assuming that this audience is somewhat familiar with at least the term psychoanalytic psychiatry and that the general outlines of its principles are not unknown to many of you. Hence I shall but very rapidly skim over some of the high spots in its developmental history before I plunge into the subterranean regions of unconscious dynamics and the resulting possibilities in aiding, abetting or producing what is familiar to all as certain types of reversible and/or irreversible somatic disease.

To trace in detail the complete history of the search for the connections between man's feelings, and the reactions of his bodily organs would take us not only far afield, but would occupy not hours but weeks. That ancient collection of wisdom, the Bible, is filled with such material. Hence if only the merest fragments of this story are gathered it must be left to your own individual backgrounds to fill in the gaps.

Darwin's conception of evolution in its general application, offers the first step in the genetic ideas which have fashioned the psychological sciences which lead one into the psychoanalytic story. In short there is a history behind everything. That history has had a development which we would like to believe is orderly and not solely a matter of chance, although we know that the trial and error method is one of Nature's methods.

Disease—in the large—is not something that just happens; a visitation from an angry god. It has a nucleus of determinism about it, a more or less orderly progress and its coming to be is, we hope, capable of being unraveled or analyzed and thus partly understood. Nature is full of compromises, of more or less stable adjusting equilibriums between conflicting forces, and everything that happens—all events—may be understood, and handled, with that degree with which the various impinging stimuli, or causative factors become known.

* Reprinted by permission from *The American Journal of Psychiatry*, Vol. 92, No. 5, March, 1936.

Read in part at the ninety-first annual meeting of The American Psychiatric Association, Section on Psychoanalysis, Washington, D. C., May 13–17, 1935.

Although Stephan Zweig essays to show in his delightful work on " Mental Healers " that Mesmer might really be named as the germinating individual of the psychical principle, it was with Charcot that clearer insight into the first of the psychoneurotic disorders, hysteria, was obtained. Hypnosis was, as you know, the technic then employed in its therapy, but of its understanding there was, through hypnosis, nothing. In fact hypnosis needed explaining. As you know, Freud studied with Charcot. In the fall of 1885—he was then twenty-nine years of age—he obtained a scholarship and went to Paris and to Charcot, at the Salpétrière. He had already done meritorious work, even as a youngster of but twenty-one years of age (1877), in Brücke's laboratory, in his studies on the " Origin of the Posterior Nerve Roots in Ammocoetes "; on the " Spinal Ganglion and Spinal Cord of Petromyzon " (1878); on the " Structure and Origin of Nerve Fibers in the Crab " (1882) and other anatomical and also clinical studies, two of which latter, one on " Infantile Birth Palsies " (1891) and another on "Aphasia " (1891), are still, in certain points, in the lead of present day conceptions in that the evolutionary conceptions of Hughlings Jackson were either appreciated by Freud or were independently developed. He really discovered the local anesthetic action of cocaine on the eye. He was well on his way toward a laboratory career in neuroanatomy and physiology and the hopes for academic honors when he was awakened from this dream by the recognition of the antisemitic feeling in Vienna's academic circles.

He then went into practice, but even as a youth of twenty-three, he was friendly with Joseph Breuer. From this combination came the celebrated " abreaction " idea, the talking out, chimney sweeping notion, which later became elaborated in the free association method which led deeper into a study of the psychological mechanisms of the dream. You all know of the early ideas of the significance of infantile sexual traumata in the development of Freud's ideas and in his History of the Psychoanalytic Movement can be found the essential details of the story up to 1914. From this time onward there has been an almost torrential mass of new research material which no one could condense within a short time.

A definition of psychoanalysis, such as " analysis of the psyche," is only a short-hand translation of a word—an etymology—and means little. A description of psychoanalysis on the other hand would explain the workings of a process and this means a great deal.

For practical purposes, psychoanalysis is a process, or method, of studying or learning about fundamental reasons for human behavior in terms of inward drives or urges in relation to the realities of the external and internal worlds. It is an empirical experimental method of investigation which can be used, not always with complete satisfaction, to learn why and how human beings operate as totals, or wholes; why they have preferences and prejudices, why they write stories, paint pictures, believe in lucky days, or numbers, knock on wood, make mistakes, get into difficulties of money, of happiness, of health, in short, a method that can be used with varying degrees of success to learn the actual manner in which mankind's mental systems operate and bring about behavior, no matter of what kind, internal as metabolic, or external as in everyday life.

It may be used thus not only as an empirical method of study, but it also has great possibilities, by properly trained individuals, of therapeutic application in the treatment of numerous types of bodily ills. All illnesses are of the " body " in the strict sense of the word. Furthermore psychoanalysis stands for a group of dynamic psychological conceptions or ideas. It is not a Weltanschauung, or philosophy. It is essentially an inductive procedure.

In all three aspects psychoanalysis stands preëminently as the work of Sigmund Freud of Vienna. Any other type of method of study, or mode of therapy, or body of dynamic psychological principles is *not* psychoanalysis. If medicine were to adopt the methods of the " patent " or " copyright " office, all other near to, or allied with, spurious imitations or distortions of Freud's studies would be infringements, imitations, fraudulent or mendacious copies. Many of them are parasitic growths, denying the parent from which they spring and which alone gives them any real validity, even if couched in different words.

The application of psychoanalysis shows, in part, that when men and women attempt to state their beliefs about behavior situations, they almost invariably tend to fool themselves. In slang terms they " pass the buck." In psychoanalytic terms they rationalize. They like to make the explanations seem reasonable. Man, including woman, universally indulges in autistic or phantasy thinking, *i.e.,* wish-fulfilling explanations for almost everything he does. Thus man's fancied beliefs that he always knows why he does this or that or how things come to be turn out to be largely fictional.

An ancient psalmist [1] said " in his haste all men are liars." While all the world recognizes that lying is a not unusual form for explanation of behavior to take, psychoanalysis prefers to use the term *rationalization* instead, meaning thereby that what is manifest or conscious in man's reason is not all that is there. What is in consciousness is in reality being influenced by something under pressure deeper down in the individual. This is spoken of as " unconscious," relative or absolute. Rationalization therefore is chiefly a compromise between what may be a real " unconscious " reason—*repressed*— and what may pass with the particular group that calls for explanation of the behavior in question. Consciousness therefore functions chiefly as an adaptive mechanism; especially when automatic wisdom is wanting.

The principle that a dynamic process of repression of unconscious urgings or drives is constantly operating in human behavior, in order to meet with real or fancied attitudes on the part of the physical or social surroundings is essential in psychoanalysis.

Psychoanalytic psychology, called by Freud metapsychology, assumes that all human behavior operates through mental systems which may be divided roughly into three parts, termed by him, the Id, the Ego and the Super-Ego. In this scheme the Id is that part of man's mental systems which has accumulated experience with the world since life began on the globe and which is present in every part of the human body. It is a billion years old and is magnificently wise. For me it is what the old Homeric Greeks meant by " Soul." Here I can refer you to Dr. Cannon's important works on the " Wisdom of the Body " (1932), and his " Bodily Changes in Pain, Hunger, Fear and Rage " (II Ed. 1929). Much of this " wisdom of the body " is absolutely unconscious. Such are the automatic activities that go on in the internal organs, kidney, liver, blood, spleen, thyroid, etc., and of the inner behavior patterns of which almost nothing is known in consciousness. This " Id " or " It," at least its oldest parts, can be said to occupy the depths of the human being. It is the core of his personality, and is that part of himself which he shares with all other forms of life, plant as well as animal. Some biologists would use the word " *instinct* " to give a short-hand term for such drives or urges that are universal to all living matter.

Out of this primitive mass of experience, and chiefly apparent in

[1] *Psa.*, 116, II.

man, a specialized part, the " Ego " arose. The chief function of this part of the mental systems is to test reality. It is spoken of as chiefly conscious and has developed words or signs or symbols, of color, sound, etc. It also is an agent in suppression and in repression. By it is not meant the popular term Ego, the self, the Me, Mine, " Mego." This latter will here be spoken of as the Personality.

An automobile metaphor may be used to roughly illustrate these systems. In such a figure of speech the *Id* is the gasoline and the engine. The *Ego* roughly corresponds to the gas feed and the steering gear operated by a conscious driver. Man's engine, his *Id,* is always running, night and day, partly idling as to outside work but very busy in internal work. In the daytime the steering gear must always be in action; at night there is comparative rest for the Ego, but the mental systems still go on operating, as frequently glimpsed in the dream.

When psychoanalysts began to study individuals with certain kinds of mild or severe sick behavior, rationalized as nervous, and also when they began to try to understand hypnosis, and the dream process, another important bit of the functional mental machinery called for explicit description. Wise people had known of it for centuries. In religion it was called " conscience." In Freud's scheme this is the Super-Ego, or Ideal Ego. It operates between the conscious perceptive system, the " Ego," and the unconscious, the " Id " and is in dynamic relations with both. In the automobile metaphor already used one can picture it roughly though not as fixedly as the hand-brake and the foot-brake. It has been built up from precept and example, from the parents and the nursery and then from the family to society. Some of it is very old but of this phyletic wisdom, as seen in reflex action for example, there is little time for discussion, although later it may turn out to be of great significance in what is called the retreat or " flight into illness."

Psychoanalytic psychiatry sets itself the problem of analyzing the respective activities in these three parts of the mental systems for explanations or understanding of any bit of social or bodily activity, *i.e.,* activity of the entire person on the environment or of the organ adaptations within the body.

The initial or primary organic or animal drives come through the *Id.* By some they are termed the primary instincts, often called self-preservation and race propagation, or what the poet Schiller called " Hunger " and " Love."

Common sense has learned and teaches that all of these factors in the mental systems have had to grow up. In infancy both the Ego and the Super-Ego are very weak and unorganized and the Id is all powerful. The child is a "little animal." It lives in a phantasy world with its primitive pleasures. It has tantrums, or sulks, or cries when not satisfied, or laughs and gurgles when pleased. It mostly sleeps. Through pain and pleasure the Ego system begins to learn about reality and then through precept and example builds up its adaptations to the world. All this is common sense. But stated · in psychoanalytic terminology, the primitive titanic Id, neither good nor bad, but just the running engine, is guided (suppressed) by conscious experience, the Ego, and still further controlled (repressed) by the Ideal Ego as an accessory brake to that degree that behavior is made conformable to the mores, in each particular situation, i.e., ideally becomes adaptive, successful and pleasure giving. In its highest form of social adjustment this adaptive process earns the term "sublimation." The forces of the Id then become socially creative and attain survival value, both individually, racially, and sociologically.

So much for the rough outline of the mental systems, the how and why, the behavior patterns, without any details of the "what," the parts, i.e., the organs, i.e., the anatomical patterns, of the body.

Millions and millions of parts are involved, but as already stated, they have had a billion years to learn their lessons; otherwise man would not be here, the fittest of all animals thus far to survive. This "survival of the fittest" is chiefly due to the generally evolving type of one organ of the body, i.e., the nervous system, and one particular part of it, the central switchboard, i.e., the central nervous system where there are some several billion central stations with dial systems of which the American Telephone and Telegraph system is as simple a sample as the alphabet is to all the books in the world.

To speak about the parts would involve much of what the chemist, the biologist, and the anatomist have learned. Much of this knowledge is necessary for the psychiatrist in order that he should get at problems of non-adaptive conduct in bodily organ functioning. Common sense knows that the major but not the only drive in the human machine comes through the race propagation instinct. All other statements to the contrary are false. One may emphatically state that neither Freud nor any one understanding his principles ever has said that sex is the only instinct in life. In accordance with this drive, however, man comes into being. The human being came to its present preëminent place in answer to its imperious urge. The hunger or " domination " instinct is insignificant in its tension compared to it. It is a supreme bit of rationalization to say that self-preservation is the first law of nature. To satisfy stomach hunger alone is a comparatively easy task, and man does not live by bread alone.

When by the psychoanalytic method the unconscious layers in the *Id* are analyzed it finds the old-old patterns enormously complicated. The chemist has analyzed crude oil and finds it contains hundreds of thousands of different substances of which gasoline is only a mixture of a few. In much the same manner the sex instinct has been found on analysis to be composed of an enormous number of elements, which have evolved from amoeba to man and are recapitulated in him in the developmental phases from infancy to manhood.

The briefest summary of these periods of evolutionary recapitulation are the intrauterine *archaic,* the infantile *organ-erotic,* or auto-erotic, the adolescent self-love or *narcissistic* and the adult hetero-sexual stages, *social* which in their highest sublimation forms evolve on through mating, nest building to a vast variety of creative productive activities.

The psychoanalytic method has tended to show that the earliest infantile patterns can best be understood by referring them to a certain content and form. To this the term " Œdipus complex " has been applied, although pre-Œdipus phases are also there. In general the " Œdipus Complex " means that since male must find female in properly adaptive cravings in order that life shall go on, the infantile models show that the mother-father images are the respective objects for the boy-girl children. This infantile model as such is usually subject to the work of repression and partial sublimation by three to five years of age. Those parts of it which linger behind in development (fixations) show other patterns out of which the " sense of guilt " and the " need for punishment " (castration anxiety) develops. Fixations of infantile models (identifications) which require extra amounts of energy to repress by both the developing Ego and Super-Ego bring about definite *character traits* in different individuals. This is but a brief thumbnail sketch of the innumerable possibilities that take place in human mental activities. Out of these character traits the various kinds of human behavior develop and become more or less fixed or habitual for good or evil. (See Fig. 1, p. 73.)

A new auto which runs along without any trouble is conceived of as O.K. and neither driver nor riders are aware of it, but when something happens, then the hunt for trouble begins. It may be within the car, it may be from the outside.

The psychiatrist then is a trained trouble hunter who has developed certain methods of research to enable him to try to locate and to remedy certain human behavior difficultes due both to difficulties

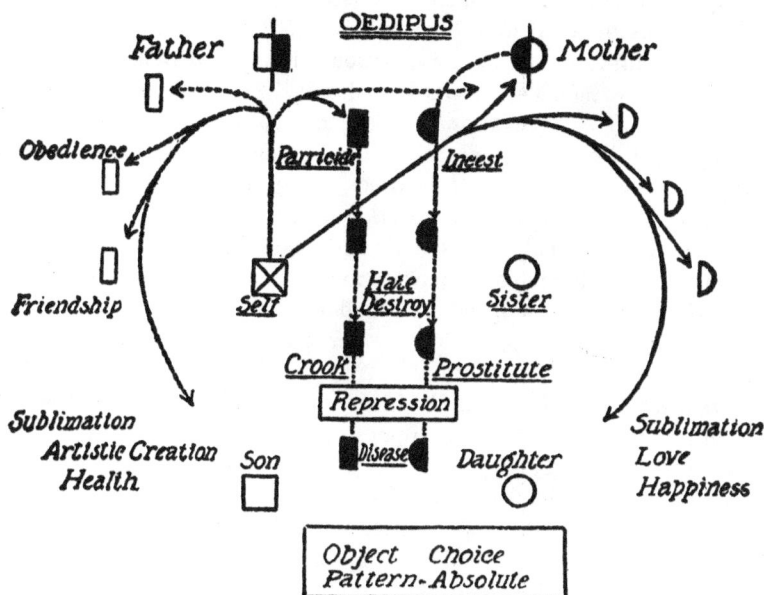

FIGURE 1

within and without the individual. He should be a trained engineer in human behavior problems and only through such a training is he competent to use the methods of psychiatry. Inasmuch as he must work with the human machine he should be one who knows such a machine, therefore primarily one with a biological and medical training. Since the most important part of the machine is that which organizes or integrates the entire machine, *i.e.,* the nervous system, he should be ideally a trained psychologist, neurologist and psychiatrist and finally since man is inseparable from his human environment, from opinions, ideals, customs, etc., the psychoanalytic psychiatrist must needs make special studies of social customs, religions, literature, and the arts. The public should know that any Atlantic City boardwalk advertiser or any newspaper advertiser or writer of popular catch pennies who calls himself a psychoanalyst is a quack.

The full details of the method cannot be entered into at this time. One should read Freud's own works, most of which are translated, rather than works about Freud's works, many if not most of which are extremely stupid and misleading.

Psychoanalysis utilizes such unconscious material as is available. Some of this material may be found in the creative activities of the individual, his poems, his compositions, his productions, his daily work. The *royal road to the unconscious,* however, is the dream life. Here free associations of dream material are most often employed in psychoanalysis. With the technical details of dream analysis we cannot stop at this time. They are highly complicated and only patient and analyst *together* in actual contact can analyze dreams. Dream analysis by mail is "fake." Other methods are illusory and much rubbish is written and talked about dream analysis.

Psychoanalysis is a specific methodology used to ascertain many fundamental difficulties, both of external behavior (conduct) and internal behavior (bodily disease). As a therapeutic procedure it can remedy many of such difficulties. Only well-trained individuals, however, should be trusted to apply it and those licensed by the state to practice medicine. Psychotherapy is the most difficult and most important branch of medicine.

Let us turn now to certain conceptions of the machine, the human being, which is to be studied or influenced by the method.

The thought which orients the present discussion is that the entire organism carries out its reactions through patterns, or purposes, or drives, or if one will, more simply, wishes. Such patterns of action are mostly fairly fixed, in part the entelechies of Aristotle, but certain amounts of adaptive freedom of control enable certain organisms to operate more advantageously than others.

All living organisms from the lowest of plants *(Protococcus)* to the highest of animals *(Homo)* may be regarded as transformers of energy. In higher forms, as in man, for example, this energy is captured by means of receptors (the senses, some twenty or more of which are anatomically known, some of which are still in humoral or primitive undifferentiated structures). This energy is transformed through structuralized bits of experience (anatomical, chemical patterns), called the organs. These activities are all loosely coördinated at humoral levels and more highly integrated by the nervous system. The energy is finally delivered through two main channels. In general, one may be spoken of as Metabolism, functioning for the automatic upkeep of the human machine, the other, also in general, as Conduct or Behavior. The chief end and aim of this conduct or behavior is the *continuance of life*.

In lower forms of life, bacteria, certain protozoa, and in certain higher forms, as in many plants, the action pattern may be carried on by a non-sexual process. The bacteria and protozoa propagate

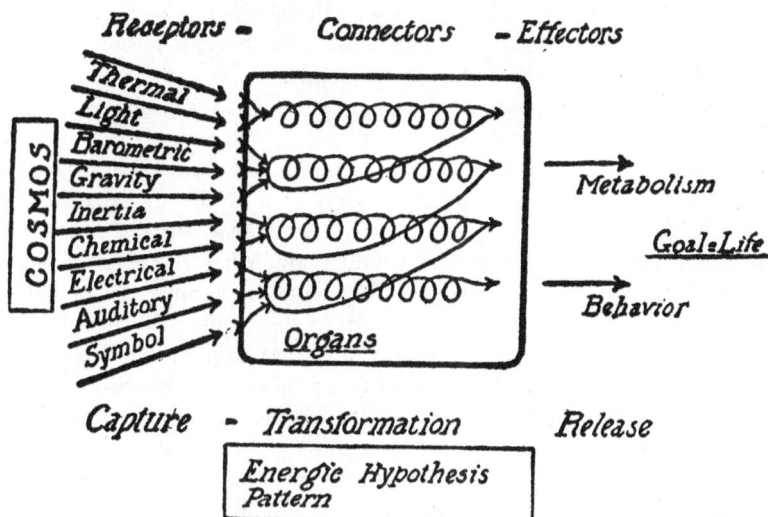

FIGURE 2

chiefly by fission or non-sexual sporulation. Higher plants like potatoes repeat themselves by tubers, or others by rhizomes and other fission forms. This type of process prevents evolution and new forms. Hence for all higher forms sexual patterns have evolved. Everyday biological science says that these sexual patterns require male and female objects, and male and female parts through and by which the living form can be continued.

The transformed energy that pursues this creative goal, either within the body as seen in growth or repair, in mating, or in family formation, in works of art or in invention, has been called *libido* by Freud. Many superficial or illy informed writers use the word libido as if it means genital activity, or eroticism or similar limited meaning.   Thus genital activities, as with prostitutes, professional or other, are not the work of Eros (libido), but of the Death Instinct (Thanatos).   They are destructive not constructive.

Psychoanalysis is only secondarily interested in epistemological problems of what is reality?   As an empirical, experimental science it makes no claims as a philosophy or a Weltanschauung.   It studies chiefly *unconscious* processes.

Expressed in a simple mathematical metaphor we can say that Conscious and Unconscious represent the numerator and denominator respectively of a fraction, in which the numerator is very small, from minute to minute, the denominator very large, a billion years. From this the proportion can be formulated.   *As from minute to minute is to a billion years, so is our conscious knowledge of what we are doing to the unconscious forces that make it happen.*   It is because of this great disproportion of the two aspects of the mental apparatus that the doctrine of " Fate " was so widely held by the ancients.

From this proportional metaphorical statement then, from the psychoanalytic viewpoint, if one would know what relationship the mental bears to disease processes in general, such must be sought for in unconscious processes rather than in conscious rationalizations. There follows as a corollary the formula that says *"Any deviation from Object or Aim (in the Unconscious), is capable of causing disorder or disaster in the delivery of the energy of the human being either at the level of metabolism or at the level of conduct, or both.*

At the conduct level, such disorders or disasters are of social significance chiefly and are dealt with chiefly by legal agencies as antisocial, criminal or delinquent conduct, or by medicine as psychoses and certain psychoneuroses.   At the metabolism level, organ disturbances result.   These are of more personal significance and are termed organic disease, acute, subacute or chronic, reversible and/or irreversible as the case may be.   Certain of these will be dealt with in our discussion at this time.

Accident must be eliminated at once.   A large number of accidents are met with in medicine, but admitting this, it is equally important to state that in some sense much chronic disease is unconsciously wished for.   It is the work of the Death Instinct.   Some of the reasons for this belief which psychoanalysis has discovered, I shall hope to point out to you.

The science of medicine from time immemorial has spoken of diathesis or tendency.   Hippocrates is full of this.   In recent years pathological science speaks of it as Constitution. Certain kinds of persons, as judged by bodily form (Kretschmer, Pende, Draper, *et al.*), are thought to be more apt to have certain kinds of diseases. This has been hinted at for centuries. The sum total of accumulated transmitted factors, chiefly recorded in structural patterns are spoken of as the hereditary constitution of the individual. Psychoanalysis regards heredity in the light of accumulated experience. It accepts it as such and to be studied by other than its methodology. The Id contains all this heredity and/or constitutional capacities. Whether all of it is capable of being brought to symbolic form is an open question. Freud regards Jung's ideas on this problem as yet purely speculative and as yet not capable of scientific proof. It may be sound intuition but is it inductive science?

The reactive capacities of the individual to the environment, internal as well as external, conscious as well as unconscious, in their entirety may be regarded as the " Personality." For more details one can consult the enormous literature so diligently collected by Roback in his Bibliography of Personality, 1929.

I would call your specific attention to what may be called the *psychological component* in organic disease processes. Other components you are aware of. (Nearly all disease may be better understood if the dynamics of the psychological component be perceived). In order to understand this psychological component it is of value to bear in mind the mechanisms of the mental apparatus as already sketched. You do not need to be told that " Life is a conflict." The survival of the fittest is a conception that needs no emphasis here. The individual is surrounded by forces with more or less fixed laws and more particularly by other individuals with their own personal goals. " Reality " is the term used in popular language as well as in psychoanalysis as a summary of these general situations. Every individual's nine months intrauterine life is a recapitulation of a billion years. This you know as the v. Baer-Haeckel law. Man is a time-binding animal. Or speaking in psychoanalytic terms, the Unconscious is timeless, the past and present and almost the future are there. All this phyletic experience is there in the developing embryo and a great deal is happening before birth, which is of great significance for the problems of internal medicine of which we would speak. This is recognized by psychoanalysis, but psychoanalysis as yet is skeptical as to the ability of its *method* to get at it. What is popularly known as *prenatal influences* are not sniffed at, but it is not yet certain that such can be demonstrated inductively through the empirical experimental methods of psychoanalysis. Psychoanalysis is a rigidly objective experimental science. It is *empirical realism* if one wishes a term of this order.

At birth the individual begins its struggle for oxygen, for food, for elimination of catabolic products. The forces of the "Id" are all important. All takes place hedonistically or in pursuance of the *pleasure principle*.

All of this has been elaborated before, but it seems desirable to emphasize the mechanisms of *repression*, of *regression* and of *conversion* if one would understand the dynamic economics of the psychological component that may participate in the bringing about of irreversible tissue changes in an organ that are called organic disease of that organ. It must be emphasized all diseases are "organic." Without an organ there would be no disease.

Life's obstacles, conflicts, which range from innumerable petty annoyances to major catastrophes, surround us at every moment. They must be adapted to. This adaptation takes place with ease or with difficulty depending upon the factors of Heredity and/or Constitution which are the more fixed features of our organization and the Personality or the more variable capacities which have developed from childhood.

The Id urges the pleasure of fulfillment of the creative pattern along individual lines. It is met, however, by the repressing forces of the Ego (Reason) and of the Super-Ego (Authority) and is forced to compromise at adaptive levels. If in the language of the energy transformations the libido surmounts the difficulties and the individual gains gratification at socialized levels, there is harmony of organic action and well being results. When only a part of the libido gratification is accomplished, and repression is, in a sense over-successful, chiefly through a tyrannical Super-Ego, sublimation becomes ineffectual, then the repressed portion of the libido pushes back to earlier stages of adaptation. The energy charge (cathexis) of the libido regresses.

What happens to the repressed libido and the repressing forces? In a crude sense it backfires, or stalls. Here is where internal medicine becomes interested. If the repressing forces are of sufficient dynamic potential to push back the libido to those stages in the individual's development when isolated organs were limited autocracies, as they were in infancy when each organ sought its own gratification, independent of the others, then the fat is in the fire.

As physicians, you do not need to be reminded how vigorously the infant will scream, as a single outlet, to signify innumerable discomforts. It is only later when by appropriate gesture or verbalization the specific source of displeasure may be indicated with the expectation of relief, *i.e.,* return to the equilibrium of pleasure.

In academic psychology, body and mind have occupied parallel pigeon holes for centuries. Down to the days of Socrates the Homeric Greeks rarely separated them. Plato spilled the beans when he " disembodied the soul," and to this day the theologians have capitalized the confusion and some have fattened on the fears of the superstitious. One of the most important of the conflicts between the Ego and Super-Ego which operates as a large factor in the mechanism of the need for punishment thus gets its great push through the sense of guilt. The working through of the threat— " Vengeance is mine, saith the Lord "—into the bodily structures is the scarlet thread that runs through the story of the psychological component in reversible and/or irreversible organic disease.

The mechanisms of conversion, of substitution and of projection as means whereby repressed and regressive libido may be more adequately managed are all operative in internal medicine problems. Psychoanalysis has learned much of conversions, as seen in the non-malignant conversions, *i.e.,* reversible processes, of Conversion Hysteria, that imitate nearly all bodily disease. The so-called Compulsion Neuroses, which in general are more malignant maladaptations than the conversions, utilize *substitution* mechanisms more particularly. In many psychotic manifestations, the projection device is manifest. Here the libido is projected from the self to the outside world, in an effort, I maintain, to *save* the bodily orgnas.

Only a small beginning has been made in tracing the more malignant and persistent conversions back into the organerotic level which can be an element in the production of chronic disease of various organs. It is premature to say *how much* of the pathological disturbance in an organ's functioning can be attributed to the economic maladjustment of repressed and regressive libido operating at the organ level. It can be abundantly proven however that some of the energy is operating to aid the disturbance. Further research with the method will clarify our formulations. In many acute attacks of eczema, of arthritis, of exophthalmic goiter, of asthma, and many other situations, an antecedent " nervous " or " emotional " situation has been a concomitant finding. Psychoanalysis has for its main object the more adequate analysis of those states so loosely and superficially called *nervous* or *emotional.* Psychoanalysis is not content with such omnibus words which mean everything and nothing. When such " nervous " or " emotional " situations are resolved into their component elements by the psychoanalytic method the dynamics of the various libido mechanisms become as clear as the respective mechanisms in an automobile with its exploding gas (Id), its transmission (connectors), and its steering gear (Ego), brakes (Super-Ego), (all crude analogies), etc.

Here, as elsewhere in other sciences, the theoretical interpretative formulations are ahead of the ability to apply the principles concretely in all cases. By analogy much is known of earthquakes in geophysics, but no one yet through such knowledge has shooed off an earthquake. Physical chemistry tells of the enormous quantities of energy locked up in a shovelful of sand, but as yet no one has been able to boil an egg with a pebble in spite of the large quantities of heat known to be locked up in the same pebble. Thus if one is to apply to clinical problems of internal medicine the principles, here outlined, while not so far off from application as are the hopes of controlling earthquakes, nor cooking with pebbles, they are nearer to specific applicability. The amount of time required for educating, reëducating and remaking the Personality is so great as to seriously hamper the worker. For the present only a beginning, although an important one, has been made. Patients, in their unconscious, resist the wish to be cured if they must relinquish some of their infantile pleasure patterns.

The understanding of the psychoneuroses is paving the way for an interpretation of the dynamic principles involved in organic distortions which very frequently begin silently or subtly as neurotic disturbances. This has been known for centuries. While in the neurotic stage of maladjustment (organ neuroses) the somatic processes are still reversible, hysterical conversions for instance, which behind a great multiplicity of forms involve the skin, mucous membrane, stomach (so-called dyspepsias), bladder, bowel (constipations), etc. After a certain number of years of such faulty adaptations (classically at about forty) the processes become irreversible. The leaning tower of Pisa has leaned too far and then " organic disease " has begun. It may be too late. *Behavior pattern has eaten its way into anatomical pattern and will not be recalled.*[2]

Even a brief sketch of some of these innumerable situations could occupy many hours instead of the limited time at our disposal. Perhaps it will be profitable to touch on certain so-called chronic disorders. Chronic is largely another word for not-understood.

Since the skin has been bathed in its ancestral sea-water-like fluid the billion time-bound years spent in the womb, dermatology offers an opening wedge. Here eczema and psoriasis stand out as two intriguing situations, still pointing a finger of scorn at current dermatological understanding. That in the beginnings one should be preëminently wet and on flexor surfaces, the other dry and chiefly on extensor surfaces, has meant little to present day dermatology; not even to allergic dermatology which entirely overlooks the vast series of problems involved in chemical cellular memories. Psychoanalysis, utilizing symbols as tools for thinking, queries in terms of flexor surface the caressing tendencies of the skin and in extensor surfaces the rebuffing or hostile activities. On the flexor side, there is taking, grasping, possessing. On the extensor side, refusing, rejecting, hitting, hurting. In these two disorders, the skin libido of such afflicted individuals activates ambivalent (bipolar) efforts at gratifications, either through autopunition (masochistic) or hostility (sadistic) repressed, regressive satisfactions at narcissistic and organ erotic levels. The repulsive acnes of many young adolescents are found to be the expression of their sado-masochistic organization. They punish their faces to scourge their souls, or they display their hostility to a kind but falsely interpreted (as hostile) world.

A very early patient with a universal psoriasis comes to my mind. Efforts at sublimation of repressed criminal tendencies through the study of law, then the practice of criminal law for relief, then additions of economic social aid for related social distorted patterns all were of little avail. Twenty-five years ago I recall I asked him, as a masochistic dream-expressed drive became certain, "Why do you wish to get in jail?" (The psoriasis was the equivalent of his intra-uterine jail.) He finally achieved this unconscious wish. It is a long story.

---

[2] Special attention may be directed here to a highly valuable and thorough bibliographic survey of the literature devoted to psychosomatic interrelationships by Dr. H. Flanders Dunbar. Emotions and Bodily Changes. Columbia Univ. Press, 1935, 1938.

Were I to stop and but briefly indicate to you what psychoanalytic psychiatry even now has to say about smell and its memories, its identifications with the body odors of self and childhood—surrounding objects and the resulting libidinal fixations, their repressions, and later regressive possibilities, I could a tale unfold about the common cold, sinus disease, epileptic seizures, and hosts of compulsive erotic reactions, which might well rival the weirdest tales patterned after the memorable classic of Livingston's " In Darkest Africa." Also were I to try to show the as yet imperfectly oriented anatomical patterns from olfactory receptors to the corpora mamillaria, tuber cinerea and the hypothalamic nuclei, I might get into psychoendocrine behavior-pattern correlations which could occupy many hours of interesting fact and profitable speculation.

For the lungs tuberculosis stands out as a striking unsolved problem. The tubercle bacillus is only a part, even if a necessary one, in the story of tuberculosis. We all harbor the bacillus. Only a few die of it. The soil that *permits* the growth of the tubercle bacillus is as of much, if not of more importance. Here psychoanalytic psychiatry has something, as yet but feebly, to say. It finds that in many instances the flight into a tuberculous disease is a way to satisfy the death instinct, either at very infantile levels, back to mother, or at more adult levels. In a manner of speaking, " You'll be sorry when I am gone," says the unconscious, unwittingly of course. Sometimes it is revealed as a form of " revenge " because of infantile interpretations of fancied favors to sister or brother or to other specially loved or favored ones. There are innumerable gradations of the " prostitution complex " of the Freudian formulation, that the tuberculous reveal. Man does not live to breathe alone. He must use his respiratory apparatus for more sublimated activities. It is not surprising therefore that the universally distributed tubercle bacillus should find an easy home in an organ which is failing to come up to its complete adult socialized capacity as an instrument of social as well as respiratory value. Psychoanalytic psychiatry can claim but a beginning in the study of the unconscious of the conflicts in the personality of those who conquer the tubercle bacillus or of those whose flight into an illness causes the work of the death instinct to prevail.

Immediately after the establishment of breathing at birth, the child begins to suck. Now from the mouth to the anus the digestive tract begins to function physiologically as well as psychologically. Conflicts between pleasure attaining and pain avoiding begin. In a sense as a child sucks at his mother's breast so will he treat the world as an object of attainment in life. It is no great wonder that the stomach should reflect conflict throughout life. It is the organ par excellence of retreat in the face of frustration. Early tendencies of the nursing infant will foreshadow many things that are to come in stomach and intestinal diseases. Constipation, diarrheas, dyspepsia, gastric, duodenal ulcers, appendicitis, diverticulitis, ileus, gallstones, maybe even carcinoma, are conditioned by personality conflicts displaced to the guts. These "diseases" are not necessarily due to the faulty distribution of libido, entirely or in part, *i.e.,* preëminently psychological, but your everyday horsesense teaches one that many of these difficulties cannot be completely understood and, therefore, intelligently treated, without a proper evaluation of *what part* and *how* much unconscious conflict is operating. To assume that a peptic or duodenal ulcer patient should be psychoanalyzed instead of being operated upon, especially after forty, is hooey. The gastroenterologist, however, *must* get an insight into psychological factors in order to be a good gastroenterologist. I deem it absolutely essential to emphasize that so far as the carcinoma problem is concerned the facts are still too deeply buried to permit even speculative suggestions. It should be said, however, that ignoring the psychoanalytic method as a part of the program of research for the ultimate understanding of carcinomatous and other malignant growths is stupid.

Chronic medicine has written a large chapter on disorders of the muscles, tendons and joints, variously called arthritis. Of late these have been more or less separated into two generally defined tendencies in which (1) joints show proliferative reactions to infections, or (2) degenerative reactions to unknown factors. The former occur in younger individuals chiefly and are now more or less officially called "rheumatoid arthritis." The latter occur in older persons and receive the portmanteau term "osteoarthritis."

For the infectious types, here psychoanalysis asks the same kind of question that it asks for tuberculosis. What of the soil, the personality, that permits, shall one say only 2 per cent or less of the population to have such joint infections even though everybody's tonsils, teeth, sinuses, intestines, etc., harbor the general and specific varieties of infectious organisms so diligently searched for by the bacteriologist, and rightly so.

Thus far psychoanalysis has only a slight look in on the unconscious pulling, hauling, muscular tensions of greed and grasping, the aggressive, hostile striking, kicking, beating tensions which are of significance in the degenerative osteoarthritides. These deep psychological conflicts are capable of involving the metabolism of the joints. They help to bring about the changes that lock up the joints in fruitless arthritic bondage when run over years of faulty adjustment. Those unsuppressed hostile aggressive impulses which in the anti-social individual forces society to lock him up in jail or hospital, in the repressed but unsublimated individual turn upon himself and through *self* punishment bring about a different kind of jail—the wheel chair. It is little wonder that the ancient theologians should have said, " Vengeance is mine, I shall repay, saith the Lord."

The analyzed cases of various osteoarthritics are but meager in psychoanalytic literature as yet. There is good reason to believe that working with massage, hydrotherapy, physiotherapy, much can be done by enlightened psychotherapy with such cases.

An interesting picture comes to mind in the person of a man of fifty whom I saw but on a few occasions professionally but have known forty or more years. He was all tied up with a widespread osteoarthritis. The X-ray pictures were typical.

If one were gathering statistics to show heredity it might be said that his mother had arthritic joints after sixty. An older sister began to develop a widespread osteoarthritis after fifty and at seventy was badly crippled.

He was the youngest child in a family of five, of which three grew to maturity. He had an intense rivalry with an older brother. There was some evidence of the older brother's early aggression. At his birth the older brother was looked after by the ten-year-old sister, this left the mother to him.

He was more gifted in many ways than the older brother but was impatient whereas the brother was more plodding. The father was a professional man. The older son studied for a profession but the younger wanted to get ahead; took a commercial course, went into business and married early. " He got ahead of his brother " he boasted to the wife of the brother. He was successful but prodigal. There were children, divorce, remarriage and widowered he lived with two daughters, one of whom had married and had one child.

This daughter was trying to get a divorce from her husband and this mix-up played a large part in the development of the osteoarthritis from the present point of view.

There was a strong father-daughter fixation and my patient, for some two or three years before I saw him, was all tied up in the emotional and economic conflict between these hostile elements. He hated the son-in-law with a virulence just this side of murder. As he described the long drawn out legal contests, prolonged beyond any possible understanding, his knotted fingers would curl into tearing tools of torture of what he would like to do to the whole situation, lawyers, judges, son-in-law, his backers, etc. " To rip out their guts " would be the mildest form of action that he would like to perform.

He was constantly thwarted, beaten, and pressed and it was in the midst of the situation that I saw him. He was not lacking in insight into psychological possibilities and after but a few talks began to mend his ways. He perceived that his violent rages got him nowhere except nearer to making himself a cripple and some few months later he showed very marked improvement although he was far from well. Economically he was in difficulties as he had spent a small fortune trying to aid the daughter in her fight and were it not for a sublime faith in his future possibilities, born of almost delusional self-confidence, he would probably be a crippled dependent. He had encouraged an ever optimistic personality to heights of ultimate success and thus the grasping at futile possibilities took the place of his sadistic, hostile muscle-joint aims with a marked improvement in their functional activity.

Here unconscious material was not available as he lived in a mid-western city, could not afford to be investigated, nor could I promise him anything more than an interesting if not profitable journey into the functioning of the unconscious. But even with the little I could say to him I was gratified to learn that it apparently had borne much more fruit than the teeth pulling, uterine cutting and other operations that had been carried out extensively in the case of his mother and sister, neither of whom had been helped the slightest bit by these radical procedures. I have the records extending now through forty years.

This is one of but many whose X-rays and histories I could show.

Many disorders of the heart are known to be of " nervous " origin. Such is the popular, and correct tradition. " Nervous," like " emotion " are omnibus words. " Nervous " to psychoanalysis means many things in which the mental apparatus is involved. They are interpretable in accordance with the Œdipus Complex pattern. Conversions, substitutions, projections and other mechanisms are operating here also. For many obstinate heart conditions psychoanalysis has proven of great service. This does not mean that rest, diet, quinidine, digitalis, strophanthin, etc., should be thrown out of the window. I should be a fool to stand here and even suggest such a thing. But even with these remedies as useful regulators of cardiac function, psychotherapy is still available even in severe cardiac lesions.

Psychoanalytic investigations and therapy finds a highly important field in the study of cardiovascular hypertension states. Here marked episodic or permanent variations in blood pressure, which often bring about arteriosclerosis, may be influenced. In many instances such vascular states are of psychological genesis which may be a primary factor which leads to cerebral hemorrhage. Straining in rage is much worse than straining at stool. Sydenham has told us of gout connected with rage and another celebrated physician of near antiquity has said that his life was in the hands of the first rogue that enraged him, through " angina." As a matter of fact he died from such a " rage " attack in an acrimonious medical debate.

The " passions," using this word in its old sense of hatred, rage, jealousy, envy and related emotional activities have been empirically known for centuries to produce bodily disturbance. The ancient injunction " Let not the sun go down upon thy wrath," is but one of the ancient wisecracks about this situation.

The only method at present known to me that is capable of measuring with any degree of satisfaction the component parts of these " passions " and of showing just how these faultily guided affective states can produce vascular and bodily disease, especially through blood pressure alterations, etc., is through psychoanalysis. Beneath the " silken glove " of " nice people " are often hidden violent sadistic impulses. The façade of urbanity may be but a disguise for intensely strong investments (cathexis) of hostile impulses. Many reformers and prohibitors are filled with such " consciously righteous " but " unconsciously murderous " impulses.

Just as any man in a regiment can get out of step, so any organ of the body is able to get out of harmony with the body as a whole. The control of the endocrine glands by the mental apparatus offers many practical problems for psychopathology. Many of these endocrine organs are very intimately related to and function as primitive nervous tissues. It is a highly significant fact that when one considers the body as a machine that operates through chemical energies, that certain endocrine organs show predilections for specific chemical substances. Iodine, potassium, sodium, phosphorus, sulphur, calcium each have their special reservoirs in such bits of structuralized experience. The many interrelations make them objects of special interest.

The endocrine organ disturbance at present best known in internal medicine to be related to psychological situations is that of the thyroid. In response to mental situations, sometimes of a very subtle and hidden nature, an increased activity with accompanying problems of much complexity and significance is brought about. Mild or even dangerous hyperthyroid states are widely recognized as accompaniments of or as directly caused by conflicts between the Ego and the Id. The Romans knew of some interrelationship between the thyroid and the uterus: you may recall they noted the swelling of the thyroid of young girls at the menstrual period and literary allusions to its measurements by blades of grass are recorded, but only in recent years has this been shown to be a close anatomical one. Psychoanalytic investigation has frequently shown some very definite conflict mechanisms which utilize the thyroid as a compensating organ activity. When this fails the thyroid activity goes on to such extremes as to jeopardize the life of the individual. Jelliffe and Lewis originally showed some very clear cases of such relationships. Many hyperthyroid states developed during the War, partly because of psychological components, partly because of altered adaptive capacity in other organs, from fatigue, etc. (adrenals, pituitary). A host of thyroid disturbances remain to be carefully investigated by the psychoanalytic method. Acute hyperthyroid states with high basal metabolic rates, it must be emphasized, may need immediate surgical intervention to save life.

"The medicine of the future," will occupy itself more and more with more accurate evaluations of the effects upon the human body of aggressive hostile impulses and with methods of bringing them to consciousness and thereby saving mankind from many crippling and devastating chronic diseases. Psychoanalytic psychiatry is aware that popular belief and theological formulations have been actively proclaiming such inherent interrelationships ever since human records have been made, whether in the form of myths, religious beliefs, rituals and observances, the epigrams of Rochefaucauld, or the wisecracks of the mummers, and vaudevillians to Will Rogers, but psychoanalysis is the first scientific entering wedge into bringing the dynamics of such human and social factors into the clear light of conscious evaluation in terms compatible with those of the physical sciences.

BIBLIOGRAPHY

ALEXANDER, A., et al.: Influence of Psychological Factors upon Gastro-intestinal Disturbances. *Psychoanalyt. Quart.*, 3, Oct., 1934.

CONRAD, A.: The Psychiatric Study of Hyperthyroid Patients. *Journal Nervous and Mental Disease*, 79 : 505, 1934.

———. Anamnesis of Toxic Goiter Patient. *Am. Jl. Psychiat.*, 91 : 521, 1934.

DANIELS, G. E.: Neuroses Associated with the Gastro-intestinal Tract. *Am. Jl. Psychiat.*, 91 : 529, 1934.

DEUTSCH, F.: Anwendung der Psychotherapie in der inneren Medizin. *Wien. med. Woch.*, 1921.

——. Psychoanalyse und Organkrankheiten. *Zeit. f. Psa.*, 8 : 290, 1922.

——. Die Bedeutung psychoanalytische Kenntnisse für die innere Medizin. *Mitt. d. Grenzg. f. inn. Med. u. Kinderhilk.*, 21 : 1, 1922.

——. Ueber die Bildung Konversionssymptom. *Zeit. f. Psa.*, 8 : 480, 1922; 10 : 380, 1924.

——. Ueber die Ursachen der Kreislaufstörungen bei den Herzneurosen. *Zt. f. exp. Med.*, 34 : 1, 1923.

——. Der Einfluss von Gemutsbewegungen auf den Energiestoffwechsel. *Wien. kl. Woch.*, 42 : 1925.

——. Das psychogene Fieber. *Med. Klin.*, 25 : 1926.

——. Der Gesunde und der Kranke Körper in psychoanalytischer Betrachtung. *Zeit. f. Psa.*, 12 : 493, 1926.

DUNBAR, H. F.: Emotions and Bodily Changes. Columbia University Press, 1935, 1938. This contains literature from 1910–1938.

——. Physical Mental Relationships in Illness. *Am. Jl. Psychiat.*, 91 : 541, 1934.

FREUD, S.: Gesammelte Schriften. Most of these studies are obtainable in English. See Rickman, Index Psychoanalyticus; and the Four Volumes of English translations published by the Hogarth Press. Robert Ballou, New York.

GRODDECK, G.: The Book of the It. Nerv. and Ment. Dis. Mon. Series, 49.

——. Our Unknown Selves. Daniels, London.

——. Der Mensch als Symbol. Int. Psa. Verlag, Vienna.

——. Psychische Bedingheit und psychoanalytische Behandlung organischer Leiden, Hirzel, 1917.

——. Ueber die Psychoanalyse des Organischen in Menschen. *Int. Zt. Psa.*

——. Traumarbeit und Arbeit des organischen Symptoms. *Int. Zt. Psa.*, 12 : 504, 1926.

JELLIFFE, S. E.: Technique of Psychoanalysis. *Psychoanalytic Review*, 1 : 63, 1913 *et seq.*

——. Epilepsies and Psychoanalysis. A Query. With F. Hallock. *Jour. Nerv. and Ment. Dis.*, 41 : 293, 1914.

——. Compulsion Neurosis and Primitive Culture. *Psychoanalytic Review*, 1 : 362, 1914.

——. Hysteria. In Osler's Modern Medicine, 1915, Vol. 5.

——. Psoriasis as an Hysterical Conversion Syndrome. *New York Med. Jl.*, 104 : 1077, 1916.

——. The Epileptic Attack in Dynamic Pathology. *New York Med. Jl.*, 108 : 139, 1918.

——. Psychotherapy and the Drama. *N. Y. Med. Jl.*, 106 : 442, 1917.

——. Psychotherapy and Tuberculosis. *Am. J. Tuberculosis*, 3 : 417, 1919.

——. Multiple Sclerosis, the Vegetative Nervous System and Psychoanalytic Research. *Arch. Neur. and Psych.*, 4 : 593, 1920.

——. Multiple Sclerosis and Psychoanalysis. *Am. Jl. Med. Sc.*, 161 : 666, 1921.

——. The Psyche and the Endocrinopathies. *N. Y. Med. Jl.*, 115 : 382, 1922.

——. Psychopathology and Organic Disease. *Arch. Neur. and Psych.*, 8 : 639, 1922.

——. Neuropathology and Bone Disease. Trans. Am. Neur. Assoc., 419, 1923.

——. Unconscious Dynamics and Human Behavior. Morton Prince Studies, 1925.

——. Psychoanalyse und Organische Störung. Myopie als Paradigm. *Internat. Jl. Psychoanal.*, 7 : 445, 1926.

——. Postencephalitic Respiratory Syndromes. Nerv. and Ment. Dis. Mon. Ser. 45 : 1927.

——. Psychotherapy in Modern Medicine. *Long Island Med. Jl.,* 24 : 152,. 1930.

——. What Price Healing? *J. A. M. A.,* 94 : 1393, 1930.

——. Vigilance. The Motor Pattern and Schizophrenic Behavior. *Psycho-analyic Review,* 17 : 305, 1930.

——. Dupuytren's Contraction and the Unconscious. *Internat. Clinic,* 41 : III, 184, 1931.

——. Psychopathology of Forced Movements in Oculogyric Crises. Nervous and Mental Dis. Mon. Series, 55.

——. Psychopathology and Organic Disease. *N. Y. State Med. Jl.,* 32 : 581, 1932.

——. The Death Instinct in Somatic and Psychopathology. *Psychoanalytic Review,* 20 : 121, 1933.

JELLIFFE and BRINK : Psychoanalysis and the Drama. Nerv. and Ment. Dis. Mon. Series, 34.

JELLIFFE and WHITE : Diseases of the Nervous System, VI Ed. Lea and Fabiger, Philadelphia, 1935.

KEMPF, E. : Psychopathology. Mosley, St. Louis.

OBERNDORF, C. P. : Psychogenic Factors in Asthma. *N. Y. St. Jl. M.,* 35 : 1,. 1935.

SCHILDER, P. : Medizinische Psychologie. Berlin, 1927.

SCHULTZ, J. H. : Die seelische Krankenbehandlung. Jena, 1930.

SCHWARZ, O. : Psychogenese und Psychotherapie. 1925.

VON WYSS, H. W. : Herz und Psyche in ihren Wechselwirkungen. *Schw. med. Woch.,* 57 : 433, 1927.

WEBER, E. : Der Einfluss psychische Vorgänge auf der Körper, inbesondere auf die Blutverteilung. Berlin, 1910.

VII.

THE SKIN: NERVOUS SYSTEM AND THE BATH *

I had fully determined not to discuss this highly meritorious paper even though it dealt with dermatological considerations of importance to both neurology and psychiatry. When, however, my learned predecessor, Dr. Bernard Sachs, introduced an historical note in his remarks, I was prompted to narrate how it came about that the subject had become of particular interest to me and why it should be equally interesting to all physicians who would escape the ironic criticism once leveled at scientists by Anatole France. *" Les savants, ils ne sont pas curieux."* It is strange how true this is at times; immersed in special problems, we tend to miss the forest in our preoccupation with a single tree or so.

When I first came to New York, young, presumably ambitious, certainly alert, the late Dr. John Fordyce, whom all dermatologists admired and respected, looking around for some bright young neurologist picked upon me to give a paper before the Dermatological Section of the Academy of Medicine, on the Nervous System and the Skin. This was my first bow in my new home and has served to keep me always interested in this relationship. An incidental note of historical interest is that Dr. Fordyce had originally intended to specialize in neurology but while in Paris his inclinations ran skinwards. As a relic of his neurological interests he had some early volumes of neurological interest, and among them he presented me with some early years of the *Nouvelles Iconographie de la Salpêtrière,* which are among the prized possessions of my library. Few complete sets of this valuable neurological periodical are to be found in American libraries.

And then as a slight companion piece to this bit of history, may I relate that the late Dr. Pearce Bailey, equally esteemed in his neurological field, started to specialize in dermatology after his graduation from the College of Physicians and Surgeons and became a neurologist.

* Reprinted by permission from the *Medical Record* for February 3, 1937.

Revised and amended discussion of paper on Psychogenic Disorders of the Skin by Dr. Eugene Bernstein held at the joint session of the New York Neurological Society and the Section on Neurology and Psychiatry of the New York Academy of Medicine, November 10, 1936.

This is not all, so far as I myself was concerned, for I recall as if it were yesterday reading a highly significant paper by Dr. Douglass Montgomery, of San Francisco, a dermatologist of international fame, in which an old Greek theme was put into succinct form. " The skin was a microcosm of the macrocosm." In spite of its mystical flavor this thought, if properly understood, is one of great significance. It means, I think, that the entire body, as well as much of the world around us, is reflected in the skin. To demonstrate this would require much ink and paper. It will not be attempted here, but a few considerations relative to the experience through which the skin has gone in the process of evolution may not be amiss.

The human ovum starts with an outside layer which for present intents and purposes may be compared with the periphery of an Amoeba. The behavior of the " skin " in Amoeba can be readily studied, as the behavior of the cell membranes of innumerable forms, both of animal and plant life, high and low in their respective kingdoms, have also been widely investigated.

In a very definite sense the " skin " is the first buffer against the realities of the external world, be they hostile or destructive, or friendly and constructive. It experiences these external forces from the beginning and must have learned a great deal. For strange as it may seem on first thought, the outside membranes in living organisms have been in touch with this external world, constantly making adjustments to it for at least a billion years. At least the geologists have told us that they find the cell membranes of low forms of plant life, the bacteria, in the earliest rocks of the Canadian Rockies, and these, the computers of the age of these rocks say, are at least this many years old.

Here is no place to enter in detail into the highly complex biochemical, physiological, and psychological processes that take place at the buffer—the cell membrane—or that collection of cell membranes, which goes by the name of skin. Suffice it to say the skin has been learning its business to survive as an organ and as an aid to its aggregate of organs, the bodily organism, for at least a billion years, and much of the wisdom of the body is its prerogative. Concerning the biochemical processes, there is no question; likewise the physiological ones, but many are in doubt concerning the psychological reverberations that may be expressed by skin structures. There is no doubt that the old Greek conception of the psyche is a correct one—namely that the " creative spirit " of Democritus, the

" reproductive instinct " of the biologist, the behaviorist's impulse, or drive, call it what one will, is just as much a job of the skin as it is of the organs of the body or of the body itself. The conception of the psyche as a disembodied soul, as it would appear was Plato's idea—and his fundamental error—has led mankind into a dualistic morass of ignorance so far as medical thought is concerned. It turned him away from sound thought and observation of the activities of the human body and of its constituent parts, even down to its electrons and protons—or what have you. Thus the notion of the experience that has been written into the skin during eons of time is worthy of serious consideration.

A simple example of some of this wisdom may be seen in the behavior of the Amoeba when subjected to the process of microdissection—a comparatively new form of studying protoplasmic response and structure. With needles in hand, under the dissecting microscope one is surprised to find that the Amoeba when pricked puts up a rather tough external surface resistance. Its pseudopodia stretch out in the effort to escape from the pricks and it behaves almost like a solid body. It might seem to be as wise as any member of a rabble being prodded with a bayonet. Moreover the interior of the cell, the protoplasm, does not alter its activity in the beginning. As the pricking goes on, however, a change gradually takes place and the pseudopodia are all withdrawn, the protoplasm becomes almost an aqueous fluid and the previously tough skin becomes non-resistant and supine. One might with little exaggeration say the Amoeba is playing dead.* It finds its external environment hostile and wisely changes its attitude, external as well as internal. The process of adaptation started with the skin and through it came the effort at reaching security by rolling away from the unfriendly darts and arrows of the microscopist's paraphernalia. One might carry on the thought and follow the skin's flight from dryness, heat, electricity as exemplified more particularly in the retreat to water, in the custom of bathing. This has been done but need not be narrated here *in extenso* since the science of hydrotherapy has so detailed a literature available.

The Amoeba began its earthly course, perhaps better its life, in the waters, many, many millions of years ago. For how many millions no one can say. The successive animals that followed in a slowly advancing evolutionary scale learned from their contacts with the waters the same kind of lessons briefly indicated for the needle

* See Kretschmer's (Medical Psychology) generalizations re hysteria and playing dead.

pricks of the Amoeba and a lot of new ones. For these surrounding stimuli, physical and chemical, were becoming more and more complex because of the fact that the waters in which all animal life then lived began to vary from the purest of rain water pools in crystalline rocks to the heavy saline seas that gradually collected, or maybe the syrupy soup as Haldane (1) has suggested. No matter in what direction one turns, the " waters " still supported and encouraged life. Hence from time immemorial " water " and " life " have been equated. But the waters have varied enormously and just as Kipling's East of Suez traveler " learned about woman from her," so the animal travelers in the many waters of life became acquainted with a score or more of different chemical substances which were washed out of the rocks which followed upon the cooling of the earth.

All the way from protozoa to man, at first through the skin proper, and then through modifications that took place in the skin, they learned what was good and what was evil. They accepted into their interiors the beneficial and rejected the harmful by methods closely analogous to those adopted by the Amoeba as it envelops a contiguous body, taking all the good out of it and rejecting the useless. The interesting feature to be emphasized is that the skin was the first tester of reality and learned its lessons long before it itself became so complicated and modified into those tucked in parts which in higher animals are called the lungs, the stomach, or even more important, as will be emphasized later, the nervous system. In other words, important testers of the chemical realities of the environment in higher animals such as are found in the respiratory organs, the mucous membranes of the mouth and stomach, the olfactory nerve in the nose, have come by long and devious travels from their original form, the skin. These later forms have lost little of the cunning they acquired when as skin in the waters of the earth they met with hostile or harmful elements and devised ways of avoiding or counteracting them from the very beginning. It would take one far to attempt to recount all of the protective devices or indicate the nature of these as preserved in the organic memory of the early functions of the skin.

When it is quoted that the " elephant never forgets," it should be remembered that bodily experience is never forgotten. Experience is written into structure and engraved—Semon called it *engraphy*— and remains ready to be used in the form of " engrams " of memory.

It may readily be argued that what one terms " immunity " and " allergy," in medicine, are engram reactions of experience, *i.e.*, chemical memories, which have been built up as protective devices through the ages and which started in the skin and some of which are still demonstrable through skin reactions.

Judging from the innumerable gadgets that nature has developed in the course of organic life, it may be stated with little fear of contradiction that struggle was always going on. To that degree that the principle of the survival of the fittest was operating, the variety of the experimental devices tried stands in direct relation to the severity of the hostile forces of reality and to the keenness and cunning displayed in the race for supremacy. Having a long time view of this struggle as seen in the light of factors that are operating at the present time and inferring somewhat as to those that have been in operation for millions of years, the tragedies in this struggle, as well as the successes, are astounding.

It is a part of this small enterprise to do no more than to call attention to certain of the successful ventures that finally culminated in man, and to touch upon only a few factors as pertinent to the discussion of the nervous system, the skin, and its contacts— particularly those of water.

As already intimated, the skin at first was a direct mediator of stimuli. As organic bodies grew in size and complexity, as they developed various bits of apparatus to push and pull matter, conquering time and space, then one and all pushed into prominence one or another type of organ or organs which promised survival values.

As most of the animals had first found sustenance in the waters of the sea, it was a comparatively simple trick of putting the sea water inside of themselves and keeping it there. This is a thumbnail sketch of the origin of blood and the vascular system, one of the earliest bits of " luck or cunning " devised by even low grade animals.

If the conception of Gaskell, the elder, be true, there arose in Silurian times a great turning point in the development of the nervous system. Already in accordance with a principle similar to that of the transference of the food supply to the tissues from the sea water outside to the blood inside, the contact apparatuses of the skin began to push their sensitive structures further and further within the body and a more or less centralized ganglionated nervous system grew. This nervous system, or modified skin, had achieved great efficiency in the insects, as in the bees, the wasps and more particularly the ants and spiders. The crucial test arose here concerning the rivalry between the nervous ganglia and the gastrointestinal canal. As the former grew ascendant in the hierarchy, the latter was impinged upon and either brains or belly was destined to win.

From the simple fact that in all of the vertebrates, but with increasing care, the nervous system in its newer development became more and more encased in bony frameworks, it is not difficult to infer how important this new device was. But even more pertinent is the suggestion how hostile were the forces that had to be met with advancing evolution. Competition became keener the cleverer the animal became. The skin buffer, as such, dropped into a secondary rôle. It was supplanted by the complicated apparatus of the sensory nervous system. They, the senses, a score or more (only morons speak of the "five" senses), now became the great testers of reality. The functions of perception, of apperception, of judgment and of manipulation need no more discussion here. There should, however, be an accent on the bipolar situation as man entered into the struggle for the conquest of various aspects of reality. Every new advance for security met with its Heraclitian opposite. Just as today larger guns on battleships stimulate the forging of heavier armor plate, the battle of unseen forces, especially those of economic and social pressures, became fiercer and fiercer as evolution progressed.

The skin of man had abandoned many self-moulding protective devices such as the carapace of the turtles, the scales of the fish, the horny layers of the mastodon or the alligator. It became less and less hairy. It has become an object of esthetic beauty and as such enters in the sexual rivalry of mate finding or rejection, of holding and discarding. Need one quote the figures indicative of the money spent for "beauticians" and their products as bearing on this single fact of sexual selection and its conscious, as well as unconscious, aggressions and hostilities in the social set-up. Vitriolic looks have taken the place of acid throwing, but the skin of mankind still greens with envy, purples with rage and whitens in terror. It even pimples and pustulates for ambivalent purposes of endearment and repugnance.

As now for many years, I have emphasized, and, as specially pertinent to this discussion, again call attention to the two outstanding chronic skin disorders which have challenged the skill of dermatologists for years—eczema and psoriasis. In very general terms, the former is more often found on flexor surfaces and the latter on the extensor parts of the body. Eczema is preëminently exudative and wet; psoriasis scaly and dry. They both probably have a number of factors involved in their causation, but one set of factors is rarely if ever mentioned in any work on dermatology; that is, that flexor surfaces are the embracing ones; extensor surfaces the repelling ones. The one aspires to caress, the other to rebuff. Here the psyche of the skin in its creative, life renewing cravings, by displacement from more maturely evolved zones of activity, give rise to the wet eczematous reaction. The death instinct of anal erotic drives shows also by displacement in the scaly repellant aspects of psoriasis. These are all hidden from consciousness, but are ways by which the skin speaks the secrets of the psyche. Dermatologists use calming lotions, as calamine, for eczema, and hostile, biting substances, like chrysarobin for psoriasis.

Another intimate relation of interest between the skin outside and the skin-derived gastrointestinal tract inside is the frequency of urticaria or hives resulting or attendant upon gastrointestinal disturbance, or even the more complicated problem of urticaria and appendicitis, and the still more intricate one, that of angioneurotic edema. As the latter has been mentioned this evening, and its possible psychogenesis noted, a brief note of such an association may be of service.

It concerned a young married man, very mathematical in trend, who before, even after, marriage had several attacks of very severe and serious angioneurotic edema. On certain occasions, his eyelids were so puffed up as to make him unrecognizable, and, when his larynx was involved, his life was in danger. Marriage seemed to help somewhat. He was, as a feeder, a greedy gulper, *i.e.,* to a psychiatric observer. At times it seemed he almost inhaled his food, so rapidly would it disappear. This impatience, or greed, or aggression, as stated was not noticeable to the unobservant. He was not a boor. I had seen him on a few occasions only, for some years, when I was telephoned for in urgency. A surgeon had diagnosed appendicitis. His wife desired my confirmation. I agreed as to the probable diagnosis, but being intimately aware of the sadistic gastrointestinal skin association, counselled careful " blood counts," watchful waiting. Six hours later, there was no doubt of the internal threat, and an appendix about to rupture was successfully removed with no after ill effects. To this day, there has been no return of the angioneurotic edema. He also had learned something about the grasping tendencies of his tucked in gastrointestinal skin. This is the Amoeba, again— the fight inside transferred outside.

The mammals, called man of this world, are filled with these grasping, aggressive drives. The World War was but a Vesuvius eruption of ever present social hostility factors which rage within all mankind. As once far distant groups get closer and closer through geographical space and time contraction, by telephone, radio, railway, aeroplane or bus, the tensions mount and mount, and the nervous system, the old skin buffer, must handle the accumulating adaptive difficulties. In the thought life of mankind are lodged the fiercest of competitive, aggressive, and hostile forces.

Nervousness is no distinctly modern sign. What is distinctive, however, is its well-nigh universal expression. The fact that half a million beds in hospitals in this United States are given over exclusively to the treatment of mental disorders, while significant of itself is of little meaning for the millions who are not, and never will be sufficiently ill to have a psychosis. And even though these psychotic breakdowns have increased more than proportionately to the population, this means little, save as a social, economic challenge, if not a changed attitude of the public towards mental hospitals because of the great humanitarian advances made in the treatment and care of the severely mentally ill. There is a greater problem than that of the psychotic, the major mental illnesses. They are the minor mental disturbances, the neuroses. The neuroses have become a commonplace. There is more falsity than truth in the apparently soothing statement that one should be glad they are neurotic; a superior neurotic, a genius, one who breaks down the hypocrisies of standardized injustices in this world, yes. But as to the minor neurotic, i.e., one who for the most part is bent if not broken by these self-same trends of injustice, in high as well as low places, most emphatically no!

How can the " needles " of the microdissection of the innumerable hostile forces of community reality of social approval be dealt with? Freud's celebrated formula of the " flight from reality " applies all too trenchantly to the innumerable " jitters " of daily life. Here the Amoeba's formula of " playing dead," while O.K. for the Amoeba, cannot be a universal formula, though some part of the device is universally and wisely used, especially in that form of a psycho-neurosis which psychiatrists call hysteria. This in many of its aspects is a living playing dead—as the schizophrenic is even less alive and more dead. Kretschmer has generalized this formulation.

The lesson taught by the manic-depressive in his maniacal flight— his alert living rush towards more living, is a highly magnified case of the " jitters " in its most aggravated phase. Physical and chemical restraint are the most widely employed remedies. Neither discharge the energy of the drive. They offer no relief for the tensions of harrowing and harassing major and minor discomforts of life. Least of all those of poverty. Here a definite return to Hippocratic medicine came in the continuous tepid bath treatment for the excitements. The psychiatric journals for the last fifty years have offered proof of the validity of the method. Before the spirochetal nature of general paralysis was definitely settled, the continuous warm bath therapy for the excitement in general paralysis was the recognized order of the day. The lessons taught by the wide use of such relaxing baths, in such severe excitements, emphasized their great relaxing and calming value in all minor excitements. The psychological effects of getting back to a primitive intrauterine fluid surrounding medium were astounding.

The psychoneurotic, or simply the nervous, however, is not a general paralytic, nor a maniacal patient. What has been learned in the treatment of these severe illnesses through hydrotherapy is of great value for the millions not so badly hampered.

To turn again to the skin and its memory inheritance. In geological terms, life was lived in the waters for the largest span of its evolution. In embryological simile, the human being relives in the amniotic waters of the mother's uterus this majestic span of its advance from protozoon to man, a billion years. This is something not to be forgotten every time one gets into one's bath and relaxes and regresses and almost, if not quite, enters into the portals of nature's sweet restorer, balmy sleep. For such is the best refuge for all the minor forms of the " jitters," the fatigues, the nervousness of much modern life.

Just what physicochemical processes are served by the warm water, what physiological activities are brought about through the touch receptors of the nervous system, and perhaps of equal if not of more importance, what psychological solace in retreat from reality, all serve to restore fatigue in the nervous system, to say nothing of the esthetic onslaught by soap on the infantile cravings for dirt.

The figures are as yet not all in and a recital of the many things that happen by reason of the temperature contact with water, with or without massage or soap, is far from being complete or final. Yet certain usually unthought of factors are of supreme importance. As already noted, a remarkable influence on the mental processes was observed in excited patients in the continuous warm bath.   •

This restoring effect has other factors than the one mentioned. The thermal factor was the one first studied since the skin is the great medium in the body for thermal regulation.

Through the blood vessels, the vegetative nervous system, the secretory (perspiration) apparatus of the skin and the hypothalamus in the central nervous system there is a constant flux and flow of influences that maintain one of the most stable of the body's activities, the temperature. Specific influences on brain function, even in its most exaggerated forms, can proceed from these thermal activities. These effects can proceed from general or local use of hot or cold water, and, in the science of hydrotherapy, many are the devices utilized to alter the flow and content of blood in one or another organ of the body. Here is no place to enter into details further than emphasizing the great influence that properly selected bathing can have upon the blood circulation in the nervous system and especially the brain (2).

Man is not the only animal that bathes, even if it be reproachfully recalled that even he, in his more primitive stages, rarely used the bath for other purposes than do many of the lower animals, namely, to drown off lice and ticks and cleanse offensive sores and dirt. Little is known of neolithic, even less of paleolithic, man with reference to his bathing habits. We suspect the modern cliff dweller, who is said to bathe but three times a month in winter and four in summer, has made little advance in this respect. One thing is however certain. His vestibular apparatus, which he got from animals as low as mollusks, gave him very definite information about gravity and inertia, even if he was no Newtonian physicist. Even primitive man could not have gone into water without recognizing that he was relieved of a heavy load. Maybe that is one of the reasons why the caves which served as the homes of man as far back as the old stone age are found almost exclusively along water courses.

Although myth making, sometimes called anthropomorphism, is one of the pet vices of thinking, perhaps it is no myth that, because of his release from gravity in his bath, something within Archimedes was loosened and the mnemic inheritance of lever actions, which were a part of the wisdom of his bones, joints and muscles, came out as the conscious invention of the " lever." Such inventions, *i.e.,* releases of billion year old experiences of the body, come from the unconscious. It may be profitable to try to correlate this relief from gravity, while in a bath, with restoration within the nervous system and surcease from fatigue and nervous excitation. This is independent of the thermal influences. The processes are complicated and as yet imperfectly understood. The general outline, however, is clear.

In the first place, one may learn from some of the early observations of Flechsig on the myelination of the fiber tracts in the nervous system in embryos that certain parts of the vestibular system begin to be myelinated about the fifth to sixth month of intrauterine life. This myelination is partly correlated with actual functioning. The " feeling of life " seems to correspond with " righting " movements of the fetus in utero.

In short, the problem of " balance " is early encountered. This is in accordance with the biological record, for when man climbed higher than the apes by standing erect, his back muscles, more particularly, took on increased responsibilities, and his two legged control of stance, as compared with a four legged table like adjustment to gravity, entailed a lot of increased special muscular balancing work with its consequent fatigue. The shoulders, the back of the head and neck, and the back record this. Even when he lies down on a Beauty Rest Simmons mattress, gravity still pulls him. But the moment he floats himself in the water, gravity flies out of the window, and muscular pull and push are reduced to a minimum. The irrevocable laws of push and pull of physics are momentarily conquered, and he is an omnipotent god who, like Prometheus who could steal fire, has conquered " Vulcan." He or she can return to the omnipotent state of the fetus in the uterus, and sadism, of the deepest unconscious kind, is satisfied. So much for a very small aspect of the psychological gain in the victory over gravity.

Reference has been made to the watery eczema eruptive state as an indication of the skin's expression of the desire for caressing. What can be more embracing than water? Hence undoubtedly the water as a symbol of the mother, of Venus arising from the water, of baptism and rebirth from the water. It has been stated how a treatise could be written on the significance of the watery embrace of the skin, not inferior to that of Carlyle's *Sartor Resartus* or Flügel on the *Psychology of Clothes.*

The neurophysiologist and biochemist further have something of importance to add to the psychological gratification.

The work of the world is muscular work. Even " thinking " is but anticipation of action which ultimately feeds into the machine of the muscles of mankind. Fatigue comes not alone from the fight with gravity in the sense just given it. It comes from the pushing and pulling of matter in time and space—inertia and gravity. Muscles, preëminently, need sugar in order to work. They get it from the liver. This is a main storehouse of a special form of sugar, which has been rendered of the right kind chiefly through the interrelated action of the hormone insulin of the pancreas and the hormone adrenalin of the suprarenal gland. This is only a skeleton of the scheme. Cannon aptly termed the adrenals the organs of "fight" and "flight." A large and fascinating volume could be written on the development of the adrenals from their earliest beginnings in chromophore cells of the skin, the sympathetic nervous system and finally the adrenals. Thus the figure of speech regarding the micro-dissection of the Amoeba, its tough skin, and its responses are repeated in the adrenal activities. In short, it starts the circuit which, as a regular and as an emergency function, begins the "shoveling" of sugar into the muscular furnace. Every physician knows that in the Addisonian syndrome, due usually to tuberculosis of the adrenals, there is the flight of extreme fatigue.

As one lies perfectly relaxed in water, the work of the stokers all along the line is suddenly reduced. Less sugar is burned, more is stored; less liver is depleted, less adrenalin is demanded. Omnipotence has come through the psychological portals; fight is unnecessary, the security of flight accomplished, and the work of restoration is at a maximum.

The warmth of the water requires less blood to the surface, the capillaries dilate, the heart action slows down, the blood pressure drops a bit, and a maximum of rest and calm is obtainable, especially with tepid or warm baths not prolonged over half an hour or about, with or without the detergent action of soap. The thinking is made easier and clearer, even when dreamy states of inner contemplation are sought. Insight is clearer and psychical fatigue greatly relieved.

Warm water works more on the parasympathetic or slowing and checking and quieting, cold on the sympathetic, the more activating, quickening and tonic side of all of the organs of the body.

Mention has been made of sexual selection as influenced by the skin. This is all the more significant when attention is directed to the matter of bodily odor and the fatty acids which reduce or oxidize from the mixture of fat and perspiration of the skin.

While it is true that there is little of the actual nosing of the human being as is the habit among Eskimos, nor is there in Western cultures any of the cow dung or human fecal anointing of the body of widows, which subserves both the principles of degradation and of exhibitionism, yet there is nevertheless a great amount of unconscious choosing and rejecting of mates on an olfactory basis.

Human fatty secretions vary enormously, but, in the main, they are more distinctive in the arm pits, about the genitals and the nasolabial folds. Indeed mothers' admonition to all boys " to wash behind their ears " has something to do with the extra fatty secretions of the mastoid regions. Brunettes are apt to have more fat follicles, and it is a commonplace of dermatology to recognize an increased bodily odor with many women at the time of menstruation, which derives from the increase in the fatty excretions of the skin. It needs no trained blood hound to trace such human mephitides. The female is not the only sinner in this connection. Certainly the heavy odor of man's middle parts can offer no easy transport to the bowers of Venus.

While repellent (or attractive) to others, an individual's odor may easily have a certain fascination for the individual himself. He enjoys his own smell. Recognizing, then, in this a motive for not bathing—a desire to preserve and enjoy one's own odor—one can understand the infrequency of bathing on the part of our modern cliff dwellers when the only reward that has been held out to them as a reason for bathing is cleanliness.

The calming effect to be gained from bathing might well serve as a more attractive inducement.

Of the significance of soap in bathing, much can be written. It enters into the process first by saponifying the fatty exterior, loosening the upper dead layers of epidermis, and finally getting down to the living parts of the skin. This is true of soap with or without massage.

This is but a fragment of the biochemistry involved. As the capillaries dilate, the excretory organs of the skin pour out chlorine in the form of the salines of the perspiration, as do also the kidneys.

There then follow a reduction in acidosis, a restitution of increased resistance at the synaptic junctions from calcium replacement, and millions of minute barriers go up on all of the sensory ingoing pathways to keep the stimuli of the external world from beating upon the central nervous system and forcing action upon it. Hence the feeling of calm and the reduction of irritability. Needless to say that experience should teach the bather that as a " punishment should fit the crime," so a " reward should fit a virtue," and baths should be regulated as to heat and length and time of the day in relation to the state of irritation, fatigue, worry or restlessness. Here medical advice should be sought especially if experiment does not clearly indicate the best effects. A very important principle here is that frequent trial will lead to better and better results just as in the kitchen or even everywhere else.

This is all very pretty, says the average doctor. One who of all the members of the community is most keenly aware of the fact that but a comparatively small proportion of the population has adequate bathing facilities. A good bath, hot water, soap, and time are mostly for the rich he cannot avoid thinking. When he reads that 10 per cent of the population of the United States pay 90 per cent of the taxes, he may well wonder what the poor man is going to do about baths, tubs, hot water and soap. Although he may have a suspicion that if many a man were more inclined to his bathtub, his water and soap, he might be a healthier, more alert and more successful person, nevertheless the social problems of poverty are not all to be solved by just his wish and his clear sense of the need.

These reflections may force upon him the conviction that no civilization is entitled to be called an adequate civilization without a free access to the means of relaxation and rejuvenation as well as of cleanliness. It is of little moment to recall the days of the baths of Caracalla and their like. These were chiefly for Roman patricians, Caesars, usurpers, and a society which in the reading of Gibbon or the like can rarely evoke the picture of realtiy. After the fall of the Roman Empire, it took a long time to resurrect the use of thermal baths in hospital practice. Charles II, King of Naples, in 1299 reëstablished them, but it is the special sign of a civilized people that free bathing facilities should be attained for all. This is true not only for the widely recognized needs of cleanliness, but to enable the known neurological advantages of bathing to assume their billion year old historic position in absorbing, distributing, cushioning the shocks of social and economic pressures now so heightened in the modern world.

REFERENCES

1. Haldane, J. H.: *Fact and Faith*, 1926.
2. Strasser: Quoted in Bumke and Foerster's *Handbuch der Neurologie*. New edition.

VIII.

THE NEUROPATHOLOGY OF BONE DISEASE

A REVIEW OF NEURAL INTEGRATION OF BONE STRUCTURE AND FUNCTION, AND A SUGGESTION CONCERNING PSYCHOGENIC FACTORS OPERATIVE IN BONE PATHOLOGY [1]

The cellular pathology of Virchow displaced an older constitutional pathology that had proved itself inadequate for lack of precision and predictability. It was no longer pragmatic. In spite of a fundamental vitality, the dynamism with which it was infused was not hitched up with the machine which the newer cellular pathology was analyzing with amazing rapidity and in prodigious detail.

The time would seem to have arrived when the vitality of this newer pathology had been drowned in details, and all thought had been lost of the dynamics whereby the *body as a whole* works. To use Bergson's interesting simile, the " intellect has conceived that minute analysis of innumerable buckets of water drawn from the ocean can reveal the innermost secrets of the tides that move that same ocean."

Cellular pathology has ditched itself in such an intellectualistic impasse and, for the most part, swung far to the structural side of life's machinery, has thought to explain its findings, either by purely static descriptions of morphologic variations, either chemical or cellular, or has carried over the worn-out dogmas of noxae in their older humoral forms. Thus the time has arrived when a new constitutional pathology has arisen which is being unevenly developed along a number of diverging lines.[2]

This paper does not aspire to encompass this newer pathology. Among the lines of development it would single out but a few—in fact, would narrow itself to one which is conceived of as the most fruitful of the newer trends of pathology and would apply these newer conceptions to the special field which this society more or less emphasizes.

[1] Transactions Am. Neurological Association, 1923, 419. Reprinted by permission.

[2] Kraus, Fr.: Die allgemeine und spezielle Pathologie der Person. Leipzig, 1919.

In this newer pathology, the " Organism as a Whole " is conceived of as the unit. It is not made up of different organs functioning as such. It is not primarily interested in the function of the bones, or the blood, or the liver, nor of the spleen, nor of the thyroid, nor of any artificial unit, or groups of units which the cellular pathology of Virchow has distorted. It would see over the top of all the so-called special activities, the individual buckets of water, and would make an attempt at envisaging what it is that gives the organism its unity, and what vitalizes it.

One of the most useful viewpoints of this newer constitutional pathology is its insistence on the concept of the structuralization of functions, particularly in their phyletic aspect. It envisages the gradual integration of new capacities for the capture, transformation and release of the cosmic energy that stands in intimate relation to the evolutionary phylum. It insists that organism and environment are one so far as the former is concerned, and that dynamic processes going on within living matter from primordial ooze to *homo sapiens* are inexplicable without the concept of this interaction.

To us as students of what in a narrow sense is called the " nervous system," this growing series of concepts is of special interest, because we are able to see how this integrative machinery has more and more been made possible through the structuralizations of a special type of tissue, the nervous system. Although many have struggled to express in some practical terms the rough stages through which this evolution of control has gone, Hughlings Jackson crystallized its main features in an apt formula. It is on this scheme that Jelliffe and White [3] have built up what they conceive to be a fairly consistent dynamic pathology of disease.

I quote *in extenso* from the fourth edition of this work (introduction, slightly amended) :

" Certain fundamental considerations are attempted in this book. It is not only a work on diseases of the nervous system but it offers a general viewpoint from which to regard all types of disease, even though it makes its main object to discuss such modification of function of certain organs as are comprised within the very broad confines of neuropsychiatry.

" The nervous system is the organizer of all experience, phyletic as well as individual, and the coördinator of that experience.

[3] Jelliffe and White: Diseases of the Nervous System, Ed. 6. Philadelphia : Lea and Febiger, 1935.

Through it the human animal is put in touch with the entire past of the race and by it can make that past of value for each moment of life. The future can only be reached through that racial accumulation of experience.

"The human being is here regarded in the light of an energy system, by which *energy is captured, transformed and delivered.* Neither as a whole, nor in its parts does it make energy; it transforms and redelivers it.

"The energy comes from the cosmos. It is caught by specific energy receptors located upon the surface and throughout the interior of the body. These specific energy receptors are numerous. The "five senses" is a simplistic concept of the truth, which has its place in the history of the development of our present ideas and the chimerical sixth sense is but a little better notion of the marvelous reality concerning the multitude of agents through which and by means of which we capture energy from the environment and then adapt ourselves to the verities of that environment.

"The histological details of the receptor structures are being daily amplified, and the means by which the captures, transformations and deliveries take place are also slowly delivering up their structural as well as dynamic secrets.

"Since life appeared on the face of the earth (estimated as being from one hundred to one thousand million years), it has unceasingly increased its capacity to continue itself through the mounting complexities by which it has captured, transformed and delivered the available energy.

"As this work is not a *histology* it cannot go into all the details of the structures serving as receptors, connectors and effectors. Likewise it must leave to *anatomy* the details of the aggregates of these structuralized functions, the organs, only lightly touching upon such intimate details of the connecting mechanisms of the nervous system as are needed for the general formulations here advanced.

"As one surveys the progress of life with a biological vision, two large fundamental functions become manifest. They are the preservation of the individual and the maintenance of the phylum. Instead of saying that self-preservation is Nature's first law, the viewpoint here formulated would emphasize the fact that the two functions are correlates, and in a sense opposites. The mystery of their opposing aspects had been the subject of much philosophical speculation from the days of Empedocles to the present time.

" The formulations followed in this volume assume that whatever is called ' Nature ' has provided for this contingency and has accumulated such phyletic memories (Semon's engrammes) as to push forward with greater dynamic potential one of these pairs of opposites, namely 'the phylum maintenance. Hence *race propagation* is the *loaded* side of life's revolving wheel, and *self-preservation* its obedient opposite. It is not a mere coincidence that theology should have phrased the same thought in the statement that ' he that findeth his life shall lose it: and he that loseth his life for my sake shall find it.'

" The biological program that worked out best was that of reproduction by a sex mechanism rather than by a perpetuation by fission. Hence it may be stated that the oldest biological pattern that successfully maintained the phylum is the sex pattern. It has been written into every instinctive activity of the phylum for a billion years or more. It must be very strongly emphasized that these statements are pertinent to the instinctive habit mechanisms. The biological conception of sex here outlined is the equivalent of Creativeness, and is quite implicitly paralleled by the theologian's God.

" From this philosophical standpoint of Absolute Idealism, man is still in his adolescence.

" The formulation in biologcal terms then states that any deviation of the inner, or instinctve habit, or good, or God-like-sex pattern will result in faulty adaptation. In what sense then is the inner, the instinctive, the unconscious pattern to be understood? Is it different from the outer, the habitual, the conscious pattern? Here again one meets with another possible series of opposites, the reconciliation of which, it is here assumed, is the chief function of the nervous system, for health and happiness by adaptation to the environment. To choose the Good and flee the Devil is the theological formula, which unfortunately, however, has so many dogmatic statements about what as Good and what is the Devil that the true Delphic formula ' Know Thyself ' is lost in the confusion.

" It is then toward a more psychological conception that medicine must look if its understanding of dynamic processes is to be better founded, and the mysteries of health and disease, not alone of the nervous system, but of all the bodily organs, laid bare. When Claude Bernard wrote, ' some time the day would arrive when the physiologist, the philosopher and the poet would talk the same language and understand each other: ' then a dynamic medicine would arise. Then the descriptive and static concepts of structural alterations would be infused with a new life and the *how* and the *why* be added to the purely descriptive *what.*

" For a long time it has been asserted that the nervous system is the means by which all of the several parts of the human unit are integrated by a species of complicated adjustments to given ends. It can be perceived how this integration is actually brought to pass by means of the *vegetative nervous system* and the chemical regulators of metabolism, at a physicochemical level, and how by the successive compounding of reflexes at the *sensorimotor level,* the human unit is further integrated, so that it can as a whole work more consistently toward broadly defined goals, the integration manifesting itself at successively higher levels in the history of the individual and of the species.

" Viewed in this way the individual is seen struggling along the path of evolution in constant conflict with an inherent inertia that would keep it at a given level, but gradually advancing by a series of give-and-take compromises that finally brings it to a better adjustment with its environment at ever higher levels of integration.

" Sherrington has beautifully illustrated this integrative action of the nervous system in the simple reflex with its innervation of agonists on the one hand and antagonists on the other, and the channelling of final common pathways for nervous discharge. This law of conflicting tendencies, pathways of opposites—ambivalence— where the final issue for higher integration is made possible at the sensorimotor level by the tension of reciprocal innervations, is found also to be the rule in the vegetative nervous system, with its double set of pharmacodynamically demonstrated balancing elements, mediated, at least in part, by equally opposed, stimulogenic chemical substances secreted by the endocrinous glands, the hormones.

" Finally an analogous ambivalent mechanism is seen working at the highest, the most complex level, the *psychic,* which determines certain aspects of conduct with the assistance of the phenomena called consciousness, in which a psychological symbolism is found replacing sensory and motor neurons, and exciting and inhibiting hormones.

" For practical purposes, then, to revert to the formula of Hughlings Jackson referred to, the nervous system may be divided into these three levels of activity, the *vegetative,* the *sensorimotor* and the *psychic.*

" This threefold division of the reactions of the nervous system is the fundamental basis on which a classification may be founded. The biological activities which maintain life at the lowest level are physical and chemical and thus that portion of the nervous system which has direct controlling influences over these activities is properly designated as the vegetative nervous system, and that part of neurology which has to do with a consideration of these physico-chemical systems because it deals with the nervous control of the viscera and of metabolism, is properly designated as visceral or vegetative neurology.

" In this region of vegetative neurology a rich variety of disturbances is found, involving the glandular, gastrointestinal, genitourinary, vascular, respiratory, muscular, cutaneous and bony system. In addition there are certain complex clinical groups involving, for the most part, the glands of internal secretion, the endocrinopathies.

" While the symptomatology of the neurological disturbances of the tear, mucous and salivary glands is a comparatively limited one, a very rich symptomatology has grown up about the vascular system in the group of vasomotor neurosis. There are many strictly neurological problems among the gastrointestinal and in the cutaneous disorders which, however, are for the most part taken over by the specialties dealing with these respective systems, but nevertheless many of these disorders will receive an adequate explanation only through the understanding of visceral neurology. Some portions of the field are as yet too little known to offer much that is of value, as, for example, the neurology of the *bony* system and the nervous mechanisms underlying the regulation of the blood cells and the relations of the vegetative nervous system to immunity and anaphylaxis, while in other systems the disturbances are known only as contributing symptoms in fairly well-defined clinical groups, 'as for example, myasthenia gravis as a disturbance of the muscle vegetative mechanisms.

" The endocrinopathies naturally form a considerable part of visceral neurology, and many of the disturbances of the several systems are still best included in the various clinical groups that are considered as due to disturbances in one or more of the endocrine glands.

" If the vegetative nervous system has for its function, in the main, the maintenance of the vegetative, that is, the metabolic processes of life, such as nutrition, growth, development and involution, the next higher level, the sensorimotor, has as its function, in the main, further integration by providing the means for the balanced interrelations of the various motor organs of the body. It has to provide that all the various parts of the machine work together harmoniously, that the functions of the various organs be not only properly timed in relation, one to the others, but also adequately related on the basis of functional demands made on them to carry out the necessary motor activities to satisfy the vegetative system needs.

" This field of *sensorimotor neurology,* including the disorders of the cranial and peripheral nerves, the spinal cord, medulla, pons, brainstem, midbrain, cerebellum and cerebrum, is that portion of neurology to which the term ' neurology ' is generally thought of as applying, to all intents and purposes, exclusively.

" The third, the highest, the *psychic level* is the most complex. Its function is no longer simply one of integration of the various parts of the individual, but at its highest, conscious level it has to do not only with the relation of the individual as a whole to his environment but more especially to his social environment.

"At this level it has been the prevalent custom to think only of consciousness, and of conduct consciously regulated by intelligence. Ideas are symbols: they are symbols of the contemplated action on things, through which the individual comes to an efficient adjustment with his environment by controlling them. The symbol therefore becomes a carrier of energy which is translated into conduct.[3]

" The ways in which these psychic symbolizations work at the highest conscious levels are pretty well formulated in current psychology, and these ways work very well so long as there is nothing unusual the matter with the whole machine. The great error of the academic psychologist, however, has been to suppose that the matter stopped here. The lower animals exhibit most complex forms of behavior without its being thought necessary to ascribe conscious motives (intelligence) to them in explanation. Very complicated activities low down in the biological scale are ascribed to tropisms, whole for man it has been supposed that *what he did he consciously intended.* Numerous studies in psychopathology have shown the inadequacy of this conception, and it is thoroughly well established that lying back of consciousness is a much larger, a more important territory which furnishes a dynamic motivation of conduct, and, in fact, that conscious processes as they are known to the individual are largely, if not altogether, determined by what lies in this region. the unconscious.

" Psychic symbols—ideas, feeling—must therefore be traced further back than the conscious level at which the individual is acquainted with them in order to understand their real significance. Psychoanalysis is as important for the understanding of the structure of the psyche as dissection is for the understanding of the structure of the body, or as chemical analysis for the understanding of the constitution of the molecule.

" The greatest deficiency in the psychology of the nineteenth century relative to the understanding of human conduct has been the neglect of the unconscious.

" For centuries man marveled and speculated and gathered observations concerning the exquisite subtleties of adaptation of plant structures to their environment. Students of Nature have recorded in encyclopedic proportions the intricacies of Nature's story of the conduct of the lower animals from protozoa to highest ape. These activities have been relegated to tropisms and to instincts. Man alone has supposed that he could explain his own conduct by reference to that which appears in his consciousness, unmindful of the millions of years of evolution preceding that which he has designated as his conscious activities.

" With the help of the hypothesis of the Unconscious, however, it has come to be recognized that the psyche has its embryology and its comparative anatomy—in short, its history—just as the body has, and, in precisely the same way as in the case of the body, this history has to be utilized before it can be understood.

" So long as the Unconscious failed to be recognized, just so long was the gap between so-called body and so-called mind too wide to be bridged, and so there arose the two concepts, body and mind, which gave origin to the necessity of defining their relations. Consciousness covered over and obscured the inner organs of the psyche just as the skin hides the inner organs of the body from vision. But just as a knowledge of the body first became possible by the removal of the skin and the revealing structure that lay beneath, so a knowledge of the psyche first became possible when the outer covering of consciousness was penetrated, and what lay at greater depth was revealed. As soon as this was done, the wonderful history of the psyche began to give up its secrets, and the distinction between body and mind began to dissolve, until now it has come to be considered that the *psyche is the end-result* in an orderly series of progressions in which the body has used successively more complex tools to deal with the problems of integration and adjustment.

" The hormone is the type of tool at the physicochemical level, the reflex at the sensorimotor level, and finally the symbol at the psychic level.

" In the phyletic history of that development which culminates in man, the symbol has been developed after trying and laying aside a great variety of tools, because it offered the means of unlimited development of man's control over Nature. The *hormone,* the *reflex,* are confined in their capacities for reaction within relatively narrow limits of possibilities. The *symbol* is capable of infinite change and adjustment, and so has grown out of the necessity created by ever increasing demands. The growth from the lowest to the highest, from the youngest to the oldest, from the simplest to the most complex has been here, as everywhere in Nature, without gaps."

With this summary of a conception, to the development of but a portion of which Kraus [1] has devoted 435 octavo pages, let us pass to the specific applications which are the objects of this presentation.

We purpose presenting a review of the neuropathology of bone disease from the standpoints of vegetative neurology, of sensorimotor neurology, both of which have been exhaustively elaborated in medical literature, and of symbolic neurology which last has been in large measure neglected or inadequately considered. Because of this lack·in including the psychic, we have emphasized the " suggestion " appearing in our subtitle, not as an exclusive dogmatic principle, but as a reminder which comes to us from a true Hippocratic principle, that unless the " mind," using that term, partly as Hippocrates meant it, and more fully outlined as in our quotation and as elaborated by Kraus,[1] be included in the intepretive program, no real adequate dynamic pathology is complete.

Lest this statement be misunderstood, may it be emphasized that interpretation,[4] *i.e.,* causal explanation, may be sufficient at any of the three levels here outlined. Inasmuch as reigning dogmas in medicine, however, have unduly accentuated the lower levels, physicochemical (infection, toxemias, chemical metabolism, endocrinopathies), or sensorimotor (nerve, spinal cord injury, neuritis, syringomyelia, poliomyelities, tabes, etc.), it is our purpose to include the symbolic level as a valuable, even necessary, adjunct, and to maintain that

[4] Myerson, Emile: De l'explication dans les sciences. Paris: Payot, 1921.

without the participation of the "psyche" certain bony pathologies remain without an adequate explanation, dynamically considered. Furthermore, it has been emphasized that the three-level hypothesis is only a general scheme of partition, the coöperation of one or more level mechanisms must constantly be borne in mind in the analysis of as yet incompletely understood situations.

Thus, as a general formula it may be adequate to explain certain bony pathologies as solely due to infections (streptococcus, gonococcus, etc.), or to chemical anomalies (gout, of older hypotheses— uric acid, etc.), as implications at the vegetative level. Adenoma of the pituitary may be, also, a complete causal interpretation of acromegaly or giantism, at the hormone level, with complicated vegetative neurologic situations still unsolved.

Arthropathies following spinal cord injury—gunshot wounds, tumor, etc.—may receive complete interpretation from the conceptions concerning spinal cord pathway function. Yet over and above these apparently satisfactory explanations, there still remain bony syndromes, carcinoma, sarcoma, certain chronic arthritides, atrophies, osteofibroses, myelomas, etc., still seeking for adequate hypotheses for comprehension and therapeutic attack.

It is here suggested that, in spite of the inadequacies of differentiation of various clinical types, without the incorporation of psychic components, certain interpretations remain inadequate and unsatisfactory.

Even if it be admitted, frankly and clearly, that following a tonsillor streptococcus infection or a gonorrheal infection, several or few joints are involved in an arthritic involvement, why the wrist or the elbow, the shoulder or the knee? Are such localizations purely fortuitous? Is such a question purely academic? Is science satisfied simply by saying it so happened?

Why is an adenoma of the pituitary? It surely is easier to ask the question than to answer it. Yet modern endocrinology is attempting to show that overaction in one set of glands of internal secretion is related in some way to compensatory relations dependent on inadequacies in other endocrine structures, either conditioned by defective constitutional endowment (whatever that may be) or other as yet unexplained factors.

Leaving for the time being this terrain of quagmires, we turn to sensorimotor neurology and really step on one of the most secure neurological acquisitions: we turn to Mme. Dejerine and A. Ceillier's [5] contribution. This work reconciles facts and theories.

"We have felt obliged to give to the first a great importance, because they are entirely new and could only have been observed because of exceptional circumstances born of the war. Also we have duplicated as much as is possible the schemes and photographs.

"We have not hesitated to give a very detailed résumé of our observations, believing that a neurologic examination is of but little value without a minute study of each symptom. We hope thus to place in the hands of our readers sufficient documents either to support or to combat our hypothesis.

"We have thought it useful, in the chapters devoted to etiology, to accentuate certain points concerning the symptomatology of spinal cord lesions, more particularly those clinical signs which permit an appreciation of the condition of the spinal cord segment related to the traumatic lesion."

Although it has seemed auspicious first to call attention to the spinal cord pathologies of bony lesions, it is not overlooked that a host of related trophic disturbances of bone have been known following peripheral lesions, as well as central spinal cord involvements. I need only mention those bone atrophies known for a long time to follow poliomyelitic involvement, and the more recent contribution of Petren [6] on bone involvements in the as yet uncertainly placed nosologic concept of epidemic encephalitis.

Thus vegetative level, endocrinopathic disturbances are clearly recognized, and sensorimotor level, neuritic, tabetic, spinal cord and midbrain (encephalitic) changes are also well known.

Involvements of bony structures, either of an atrophic or a hypertrophic nature, due mainly to complicating psychic factors, have been largely overlooked. These have been recognized and have appeared in neurologic literature from time to time. This is well appreciated, but inasmuch as the medical disciplines have had a definite tendency to ignore them and have attempted to subordinate them to conceptions of a more simplistic and mechanistic nature, we have here been inclined to emphasize them.

As indicated, the rearrangement of endocrinopathic and vegetative bony syndromes, and of the sensorimotor syndromes is to be pre-

[5] Ceillier, André: Para-ostéo-arthropathies des paraplégiques, par lésion de la moelle épinière et de la queue de cheval. Paris: Lahure, 1920.

[6] Petren, K., and Brahme, L.: *J. Nerv. & Ment. Dis.*, 57: 105 (Feb.), 1923.

sented in more extended form, and we here pass on to the consideration of the special case which is used as an argument pertinent to the need for a study of psychogenic factors if a more complete understanding of bone pathology, in certain cases, is to be obtained.

REPORT OF CASE

Clinical History.—Mrs. M. D., white, aged forty-two, who had been married sixteen and one-half years, was seen Jan. 11, 1921. The hereditary and personal history are without significance. She began to menstruate at thirteen; and has two children, aged fourteen and twelve, respectively. She has had some more or less persistent leukorrhea since girlhood.

In 1916, she did a lot of war gardening and fatigued herself markedly, and soon thereafter noted that she had vague distress in the left leg near the ankle which caused her to favor this leg and thus began a slight limp. Her first physician gave her foot plates. A second orthopedist said no plates. A third said her leg needed developing. In 1919, another orthopedist said she needed exercises. She took them. They were very painful and she did not recover. Then a diagnosis of an hysterical limp was made and confirmed later after a second neurologist's examination. On the recommendation that she needed psychotherapeutic treatment she was referred to me.

Neurologic Examination.—My first neurologic examination was not conclusive. The cranial nerves were healthy but hyperexcitable and there was a doubtful Chvostek sign. The upper extremities showed no anomalies save marked hyperexcitability of the skin and tendon reflexes ($+++$, and $++++$), definite hypertonus and fine static tremor of the neck, arms, trunk and fingers. The reflexes of the lower extremities were equally hyperexcitable.

The knee jerks were $+++$ with slight predominance of the left side. No clonus was obtained; no Babinski sign was elicited, yet the flexion response of the left side was definitely diminished. The achilles jerks were active ($++$), the right definitely more marked than the left. There was slight disturbance of epicritic sensibility to touch in the left leg and foot. There was definite diminution in size of the leg—¾ inch—at the gastrocnemius level, and slight reduction in size of the left thigh ½ inch. These atrophies had been noted by one examiner.

With reference to the almost spasmophilic type of reflex response, she detailed that at times she had noted that even if she was lightly brushed against while sitting she would jump.

Focusing attention on her gait, I observed she was very tense and trembly, her face would almost flush, the pupils dilated and the skin became moist. " She hurried from the left to the right foot." This was a true description provided by one of her orthopedic surgeons. I inferred some definite protopathic pain focus and asked for a roentgenogram of the leg before further investigation.

This report was disconcerting. The roentgenologist reported a myeloma. Urinary examination and extensive roentgen-ray examinations of other bones followed. No Bence Jones proteids were present, and there were no multiple foci; the roentgen-ray diagnosis was modified to cystic formation of large benign giant cell sarcoma type. There was moderate anemia. I counseled conservative treatment, telling the husband it was a surgical condition, but that the concensus of opinion among surgeons (Colby, Codman and others) was to follow conservative measures in this type of condition.

Focusing attention on the spasmophilic condition, I proposed, after full discussion, a research to see if any psychologic factors might throw light on her extreme " nervousness " which has led in the first place to the belief in a " functional limp." This suggestion was accepted and accordingly I started a psychoanalysis. The full details of this analysis are not pertinent here.

The first dream showed definite regressive tendencies: " *I squeezed through a hole in the fence in the churchyard. The janitor put me out. Then a brother-in-law was beating his wife and the children were crying. Then the sister and I again went through into the churchyard and again we were put out. A brother-in-law walked through this small opening, then I turned to the keeper and jokingly said I was so thin I could squeeze through such a small opening.*" To the psychoanalytic worker the unconscious suicide wish in this dream was suggestive and I was intrgued to find out what it signified.

A second dream opened up an annoying situation in which a trained nurse who had wormed herself into the family had finally been ejected, and there were distressing threatened legal worries.

After about a month of analysis there came clearly into vision an interesting " sleep ritual " which was found to have persisted many years. The patient could not sleep until the left leg was tightly pressed against the right, the left foot lifted over the right and held in a strongly inward rotated and extended position. How many years this had been going on she was unable to say, but at least a year later, at a later period of analysis this leg-foot position was brought into definite correlation with a left-hand posture associated with violin playing as a girl. She had great difficulty in getting her fingers sufficiently far over the strings of her violin and for some years her teacher upbraided her. In this strain for a finger-wrist position she recalled a compensatory leg-ankle position. The harder she strove to get her wrist and fingers flexed, adducted and everted, the more there was a corresponding adduction, extension and inversion of the left leg. What lay behind this was unknown.

Early in the analysis it became apparent that there were some definite repressions at work which interfered with complete satisfaction in coitus.

These showed that the leg-foot position was functioning for at least two ill-defined goals. In the first place, the adduction of the thigh was unconsciously symbolized as a protection to the entrance of the vagina. It never reached the stage of dyspareunia, but the dissociated component in the unconscious revealed that the husband was a dual being, mostly acceptable, but partly rejected because of identification with a polygamous possibility (father imago). This had made the orgasm an almost unattainable goal, notwithstanding intense excitement and consequent frustration.

The second unconscious goal attained by this sleep ritual was to bring the labia together to obtain unconscious masturbatory satisfaction.

Following the uncovering of this general situation, the patient made a striking readjustment. She lost nearly all her tenseness. The reflex excitabilities disappeared. She realized the futility of her self-destructive attitude and came into far better rapport with the husband. This showed itself in consciousness by the easier attainment of the orgasm, with less effort and great relaxation. The spasmophilic situation disappeared entirely, she became philosophic, and things which had incessantly worried her she threw off with equanimity. "I should worry!" became her slogan and she was much happier. She gained some 20 pounds and reached the weight of 140 pounds. The roentgen-ray findings after the first six months of observation, however, were progressive. There was also a progressive secondary anemia. Earlier records, 1919, showed the hemoglobin 78 per cent. In January, 1921, when I first saw her, the hemoglobin was 74 per cent. In May, I prescribed parathyroid substance, ¼ grain (0.016 gm.), and did not see her after June until the following January, 1922.

The roentgen-ray report was as follows: "The process is no

more extensive; that is, it does not involve more of the shaft of the bone than it did at the previous examination, but there is more definite evidence of a tendency toward a cystic development or loculation than there was at the time of the previous examinations. The rather large loculations observed at this time are more suggestive of the giant cell type of sarcoma; there is more evidence of a crushing, impaction and deformity of the inner malleolus, and the tilting of the astragalus resulting from this impaction is more marked. I believe, therefore, that the process is definitely progressing."

In view of the progression of the tumor formation, and believing that at least a vicious circle had been established, I prescribed roentgen-ray treatment. I, however, continued my analysis.

The record of the roentgen-ray treatment is:

Jan. 31, 1922: 200 kilovolts; time, 40 minutes; distance, 30 cm.; milliamperes, 3; filter, 0.5 cm. copper and 2 mm. aluminum; anterior aspect of left lower leg.

Feb. 7, 1922: 200 kilovolts; time, 40 minutes; distance, 30 cm.; milliamperes, 3; filter, 0.5 cm. copper and 2 mm. aluminum; posterior aspect.

The roentgenogram of March 7, five weeks after treatment, showed no improvement.

April 5, another roentgen-ray treatment was given: kilovolts, 200; distance, 50 cm.; time, 4 hours; milliamperes, 3; filter, 1 mm. copper and 2 mm. aluminum. Left lower leg anterior, lateral, external and lateral internal aspects.

May 17, 1922, another roentgenogram was taken, with the following report: " The condition is practically the same as at the previous examination. There may possibly be a slight increase in the breadth of the articular surface of the lower end of the tibia—a ' flattening out' process. There is a slight increase in the bone salts along the inner border of the tibia and internal malleolus. The cystic degeneration is practically the same. There has been no extension up the shaft of the bone. The process has all the characteristics of a giant cell type sarcoma, which is non-malignant."

Psychoanalysis was continued from January to June, 1922. Nothing was done during the summer, save blood examinations which showed betterment of the anemia.

A roentgenogram was taken Dec. 6, 1922, about two years after the first visit. The report of the radiologist follows:

" In comparing these films with those made at the last examinations, there is definite evidence of the increase in density in the area affected. This is most marked in the tibia and is probably due to the increase in fibrous tissue throughout the affected area. The deformity, that is, the tilting of the articular surface of the astragalus, is about the same as at the former examination. There has been no extension of the process and one is justified in stating that there is definite improvement in the area affected."

From February, 1923, to the present time I have seen her about once a week. During these sessions a number of relevant situations of psychoanalytic interest were brought out, only one of which was significant. This seemed to bring into the foreground the origin of the vulvar masturbatory activity. I will not be dogmatic on this as I have not enough evidence, but it seemed to be shown that in the effort of the patient at the age of nine months to control her bladder, she had learned that labial pressure aided her, but the dream material might be interpreted to indicate that at the same time she found a pleasurable erotic gratification by the self-same maneuver. It had been definitely proved that this type of labial pressure was an infrequently resorted to activity, partly unconscious, partly conscious, in order to satisfy the onanistic gratification, recognizable as such from at least the age of fourteen or fifteen, at which time consciousness of the leucorrheal discharge arose. I therefore conjecture the persistence of the old mechanism and argue its importance in the dissociation of genital activity in the marriage relation.

Summary

A rapid summary of the suggestive reasoning relative to the localization of the pathologic process, if not its origin, would be as follows:

The gradual development of a postural muscular tension with the outlined unconscious psychic goals. This postural tension, because of the unconscious motivation, was a chronic one. This entailed at least two types of activity: (1) Constant afferent and efferent nerve pathway activity with general signs of fatigue (spasmophilic reaction-calcium-parathyroid mechanism disturbance). With this mechanism in view, attention is directed to certain available data concerning the innervation of muscular and of bone components. (2) I am disposed to direct special attention to the study of the anterior annular ligament and the tibio-astragalar ligamentous connections.

I find no kinetic observations which will enable me to state in definite terms the amount of strain that was constantly operative on the anterior annular ligament in the maintenance of the posture which I have described. Anatomists consulted stated it to be definite, and I postulate on the basis of this a constant periosteal irritation over the area of insertions of the anterior ligament.

On the basis of (1) chronic fatigue of afferent and efferent radicular nervous activities chiefly involving the tibia so far as bony response is concerned (atrophy of muscles as well), and (2) local continuous irritative phenomena through ligamentous periosteal activities, there resulted a serious imbalance of metabolic stimuli in the area involved. Atrophy with secondary cystic formation took place, *i.e.*, the so-called non-malignant cystic giant cell sarcoma. At this time I am only secondarily interested in the classification of this formation. My chief interest has been to try to learn if a neuropathologic situation, with predominant unconscious psychogenic factors might not offer an insight into dynamic mechanisms affecting bone metabolism.

IX.

PSYCHOANALYSIS AND ORGANIC DISORDER: MYOPIA AS A PARADIGM [1]

Keyserling in his *Travel Diary of a Philosopher* [2] states, " For man is not only man, he is simultaneously, in various parts of his being, animal, plant, rock and sea; only he rarely becomes conscious of the fact and only knows how to feel as a human being."

No matter how many times down through the centuries this general concept of mnemic binding of external contacts through internal integration is expressed, now in one form, now in another, the essential unity of outside and inside relationships remains an outstanding bit of reality.

As one traverses the world we live in with this genial philosopher in this self-same *Diary,* one is uncertain whether most to be struck by the richness of the objective manifestations detailed, or to marvel at the ingenuity of penetration of the internal subjective concentrations suggested.

Glimpsing through the innumerable fascinating vistas opened by Keyserling one is impressed again and again with the general plan of *bipolarity* underlying all the external and internal manifestations which have come under his observation, and, as an aside, just as he counsels a year's stay in Benares for those who would wish to get into the inside of the religious experience, and a year's compulsory residence in China for our self-sufficient men in ethics and morals, so, in this same spirit of counsel, I can conceive of no better suggestion to the psychoanalytic student than to travel once at least around the world and study deeply the bipolar types of expression of the human organism. [3]

As, from the objective point of view, the macrocosmic canvas will never be big enough upon which a colossal industry will be able to

[1] Shortened outline of Communication given at the Ninth International Psycho-Analytical Congress, Bad Homburg, September, 1925. *International Jl. Psycho-Analysis,* 7: 445, 1926, from German original, *Int. Ztsc. f. Psa.,* 12: 1926, Heft 3. Reprinted by permission.

[2] Vol. II, p. 144, English edition.

[3] An interesting contribution to this thought is Alexander's " Der Biologische Sinn psychischer Vorgänge," *Imago,* Bd. IX, 1923, in which the Buddhistic inner experiential or intuitive methods are discussed psychoanalytically.

paint the doings of humanity, so also from the subjective point of view—the microcosm—no microscopic eye will ever be able completely to refract into its integers the masterly accumulations within the individual of Nature's experiences with that self-same Cosmos. Fortunately the psychoanalytic method does justice to this bipolarity, and East and West may ultimately be shown to be at one if their ambivalent factors may be reconciled.

Drawing closer to the subject of my paper, first from the objective point of view—and limiting this view to the small, yet vast group of phenomena in medicine termed myopias—permit me to say that I would essay a purely tentative, I might more rightly say, a purely speculative approach. Speculative in two senses—one as in accord with the general logical thesis that all studies along the lines contemplated can hardly be termed more than a series of speculations at best, and second, a personal acknowledgment of a somewhat cursory effort in the specific direction of the inquiry suggested.

Still further I purpose focussing attention upon one group of the myopias, the which, however, ophthalmological science recognizes as showing a fairly constant phenomenology.

The congenital myopias are rare. These will not concern us—nor those apparently acquired in the early years of infancy, also, numerically speaking, insignificant. The group to which attention is here drawn is that which bulks large in ophthalmological experience and which temporarily clusters about the puberty period—viewing this period with the wider ranges of extension which analytic research has shown it to possess. These myopias then which are more or less rapidly determined from ten to eighteen years of age, but with apical supremacy in the incidence curve from fourteen to sixteen years of age, and shading off as indicated. Phenomenologically, these myopias are noted more particularly in boys and girls as they are in their high school or early college period. The myopia is usually attributed to some special applicatioin in reading, or, in girls, doing fine needlework or something of that general nature. It advances slowly within 1–2–3 years to degrees of 2–4–6 and more diopters. Glasses are prescribed, changed a few times, and the series of changes apparently cease; the myopic norm is established and remains so more or less throughout life.

From the descriptive somatic side ophthalmological science chiefly accents the lengthening of the optical axis by elongation of the eyeball. It has measured this in innumerable instances and most frequently focuses its attention upon the external muscles which pull the sclera and thus deform the instrument. Certain studies deal with sclerical changes as permitting this deformation. Only within recent years has the vegetative nervous mechanism present in involuntary muscle been interrogated as playing a rôle in this new adaptation.

Another factor, which, so far as may be definitely stated, may be involved, but as yet lacks the measurement exactness of that just recorded, is concerned with the internal muscles of adaptation acting upon the crystalline lens. Here sthenic or asthenic muscular reactions—using those older bipolar terms of tonal support—are undoubtedly involved, although as stated, ophthalmological science—the which I cannot claim to have exhaustively searched—still lacks precise formulation.

Reduced to simple terms, which may however conceal more than reveal, we are dealing with an effort syndrome which elongates the eyeballs and which tends to increase the convexity of the lens.

The histological changes which parallel these larger findings cannot be entered into here, although they ultimately must be correlated in a causal relational pathology.

Viewed from an obvious psychical platform two questions may be asked. Since far vision is lost and near vision in a sense enhanced, what large environmental contact is the individual seeking to eliminate from visual perception in order to concentrate upon a smaller world of optical reality? Or viewed from an inner platform or panel, speaking in terms of relational frames, what purpose or wish-fulfillment, in its most general sense, is being pursued?

This is the kernel of our inquiry. The answer, here postulated and toward which some confirmatory evidence is offered—a castration symbol.

It is in but a minor sense that the conception is here regarded as new or novel, since I take it that it has been so often stated by others, and not infrequently emphasized by Freud whom we all take pleasure in honoring as having offered more explicit intellectual tools to prove that which intuitively has been glimpsed for centuries.

Thus St. Paul's pronouncement has been chosen as the central theme of this intuitively arrived at formula: " If thy right eye offend thee, pluck it out." The mystics' meaning of " offense "—as well as the " means " by which the relative destruction has taken place—may be opened up by the psychoanalytic discipline and the " symbolic " truth reduced to rational terminology in terms of a dynamic pathology, and ultimate therapeutic relief of a different type than the wearing of glasses, which after all must afford but a partial compromise with the inner conflict.

Innumerable considerations, possibly of absolute value in a strict logic, are here pushed aside, conditioned by individual insufficiencies, or temporal considerations, but chiefly because of the purely preliminary nature of this presentation. I can present but a moiety of the numberless torsos of observation which have passed before my eyes. I cannot claim to have as yet satisfied my own canons of sincerity of exhaustive research. The majority of the observations have been extremely fleeting and belong to a crude natural history— a few have been more fortunately offered for more detailed study, and as yet but tiny fragments of psychoanalytic research—but even so, with the crudity said to so persistently stamp the cultural processes of the far West, I have the temerity to offer them.

One of my keenest and ablest students, a youth of eighteen, when I was a young teacher of pharmacognosy of thirty, was a pronounced myopic of the type under consideration. The explanation offered was the banal one of over-application to interest in intellectual pursuits with the added factor that he would read into the night with candlelight in order to avoid his father's prohibition of his reading after a legitimate retiring limit. I have known him thirty years at conscious levels, but my first faint questionings of the myopic problem began with the observation of this general type of cultivated, eager, studious intellectual kind of person which seems to bulk large in the ophthalmological literature of myopia. Dimly I have caught glimpses of his inner problems, through his young married life, early widowhood, with tragic loss of his life partner—possibly a not unrelated bit of social pathology—his later scholastic and academic career, his friendships, and a diabetic later development—which point in the general frame of some narcissistic fixation factors—the whole, logically considered, if presented as a bit of science, would afford a Gargantuan opportunity for caricature of psychoanalysis. Yet here I am willing to be an impressionistic novelist of the most speculative stamp.

Early in my psychoanalytic period, a most pronounced example zigzagged through my consultation room. A young woman of about thirty who, beginning as the type formulated, had by virtue of exaggeration of inner conflicts, pushed her myopia up year by year until it had reached the preposterous grade of 20–25 diopters. She was a malignant, as contrasted with the benign type just hastily sketched. Eccentric, wild, exaggerated, self-willed, musically talented, discontented, the few hours' contact brought into sharp outline an almost catatonic personality which threatened to disrupt at any moment, but the which, I take it—in all humility—was prevented by the masochistic self-destruction, through the eye-relationship with reality. Here the homosexual repressed factors were obvious even to the psychoanalytic tyro I then certainly was. Here again, impressionism is all that I can legitimately offer.

Another sample, more exhaustively studied, may finally be considered. It, like so many of the problems in the borderland of somatic and psychopathology, was not studied from the standpoint of our title. Very few patients come to be studied for these types of irreversible organic disease or deformity, and hence, like many another study conducted upon skin, bone, blood, heart, lung, kidney, eye or ear pathology, the patients have come for relief for some difficulty to them more pregnant with meaning, and only as incidental to my therapeutic work have I been intrigued to make occasional forays into the psychosomatic relationships which are universally present and which some day may be regarded as Hawthorne has so succinctly stated in his *Scarlet Letter*, "A physical disease which we consider as something separate and apart, may be after all but a symptom of disorder in the spiritual part of our nature."

This patient, a young business man of relatively healthy and sound ascendants, was thirty-one years of age when first seen. He had a married sister of thirty-five, an unmarried sister of thirty-three, and a younger married brother of twenty-nine. He looked after the property interests of a prosperous professional father, integrating them into a larger business activity. He read early, had an exclusive private school and college training, was a rower and developed into a tall, strong, attractive American type of bachelor. In spite of all this good physique and active participation in sports, etc., he remained quiet, somewhat retiring, even timid, and came for consultation and possible treatment because of his inability to push himself, reluctance to be a " go-getter," timidity and fear of women and an annoying tendency to blush, particularly in the presence of women, but also in the presence of men.[4] He had never been in love, was apprehensive of marriage, and although no conscious purist or puritan, his actual erotic relations with the *demi mondaine* were conditioned upon a special bit of conduct.

⁴ Benedek, Th.: " Aus der Analyse eines Falles von Erythrophobie." *Int. Zeit. f. Psa.*, Bd. II. 1925. 88.

He had to drink. When well liquored his entire personality underwent a very definite change. From being retiring and quiet and more or less terse and apodictic—saying yes, and no—and being a listener rather than a talker, he became highly sociable, was witty, and even a most entertaining comic artist. He became the life of a party and would extemporize poetry, became a great raconteur, and wooed women, of a complaisant type, with great interest and success. He practically never sought them by himself but always went along with the crowd and had a great time. With "good" women he was always on guard, and unless well alcoholized, even under the most auspicious surroundings, was impotent.

So far as our theme is concerned, his general analysis cannot be entered into; his myopia began when he was in prep. school, about twelve to fourteen. Masturbatory activities had a spurt about ten, were feared and suppressed and then later accepted with some struggling repulsion. Cohabitation began at twenty-one and under circumstances mentioned; this latter situation had remained as outlined up to a certain period in the analysis.

The myopia advanced slowly, and by his second or third year in college, eighteen to twenty years of age, was fairly stable. He had about four or five diopters. He could distinguish people in the immediate environment without his glasses, but was not certain as to their features.

Our analysis began about the middle of February. From the first the dream material was ample although associations have not become "free." The first dream may be recorded. It was of interest in view of the behavior alteration under the regressive influence of alcohol. *I am at a stag dinner. All is quite convivial. A man arose to speak. No one paid any attention to him. He finally got up on top of the table and walked up and down on it. Rather queer, I thought, his soiling the tablecloth that way.*

Its partial analysis naturally brought out much of the material alluded to as his activity when having a good time in male company. It evidences, I take it, certain aspects of repressed hemoerotic components which are not without importance in his general analysis.

The second dream two days later led directly into the Œdipus situation. *I am somewhere with my father. We meet a woman, she is married and she said that her husband had died. She was making a wreath of flowers for his grave. I wanted to talk with her but my father monopolized her attention. He finally sent me off to close a couple of doors of a closet.* [Vaguely familiar, like those in the house where I was born.]

This general Œdipus conception was quite readily accepted, intellectually, but it remained repressed emotionally. It seemed quite logical to the patient, and his general family neurotic romance situation was quite conscious in its features as Rank has outlined them.

The discussion of the dream lead directly to a week or two of resistance and negative transference defensive dreams which were very passively handled. These do not need recital here, as we are now more concerned with the entrance into the dream symbolism of his eye situation—even though it is recognized that such a separation of the material is purely arbitrary. These resistance features slowly were building up a " father-brother " identification pattern. In a dream of March 6th, I appeared in the dream—*sitting on a chair next to him in a club locker room. You were my age.* He did not want to join a club to which I belonged—some discussion about it! A " sight " feature here appeared for the first time, *something was written on a large bulletin board—Article on Physical Culture Type of thing. Care of woman before childbirth. In white chalk—something about a sac, which burst with a loud report—other unknown details.*

Infantile peeping and even adolescent peeping memories were very definitely covered and under repression—partial analysis here showed. Amnesia was profound then and still remains.

March 16th: Dream of last night mostly gone. *" I broke my glasses. I was looking in some basement dining room, several girls were there [inside sitting-room]. In some way I got inside and was talking with a girl. I think I asked her to dance. I dropped my glasses. At first the lens only cracked, but as I started to straighten them out, they broke [right glass only] in three pieces—I could not see so well then."*

This dream started a few inquiries regarding his myopia. One eye was worse than the other—which one he could not recall [right in reality].

No peeping material came out of the associations and no memories were evokable. Interpreted as resistance material. Also to myself were the first intimation of the castration complex shown early in the father prohibitions—conscious fear of father and slight anxiety in his child and adult contacts with him—very fond of him but quite distant. Rarely likes to enter into any discussion—which is often quite necessary in view of close business association—" always uses the mother as an intermediary ".

The relation between his right broken lens and his castration with the girl (dancing) perhaps hardly needs emphasizing in this assembly. Associations permit certain inferences binding the alcoholic perceptive cloudiness with the optic perceptive cloudiness and the incest prohibition barrier—sister, just older—is beginning to emerge as the mother—displaced libido carrier.

If I can't see, I do not know (mother-sister) hence I may possess (mother-sister) and get past the barrier—impotency=alcoholic reduction=eye reduction. Impotency is overcome with (inferior—superior) servant girl—sister (demi mondaine cohabitation) when full of booze.

March 8th: Hetero-homosexual identification. Girl becomes man. Height—seeing proposition.

March 10th: *I am in a department store and wanted to go downstairs in the elevator. As I moved towards it I saw on the counters a lot of babies displayed instead of the ordinary goods. I entered the elevator, it was very wide. Other people also in it. A man called out his floor; on that floor there were a lot of Mercedes cars stored, as in a garage; most of the people got off. I also got off but decided to go on down with the elevator, which now seemed separated from the floor by a gap, undecided and anxious and finally jumped on the elevator. Another man was in the uncomfortable position of straddling the gap. I finally gave him a hand and pulled him on.*

Associations: The thought of the babies annoyed him—each one had a nurse—then the nursery activities were very repugnant, especially wet clothes, bed clothes, games of hiding under the bed clothes.

Anxiety was most marked about making the gap. Not so hard after all when he made it. Also was able to help the other man quite readily. This is a very characteristic feature of his business reluctance. He holds back and holds back, but once started, sometimes by a little shove from some outside source, and it becomes very easy after all. All but the interest in a woman.

He only saw the back of the elevator man. The people who mostly disappeared at this Mercedes floor were men. Only one woman. Quite indistinct.

The autos were Mercedes cars, large expensive fast cars, foreign cars, exhibitionistic—bruiser type—real estate mortgages—title insurance—certain type of business man—know it all—Father—the whole auto situation was certainly his father. He had feared him all his life—anxiety quite of that type—every once in a while he had experienced quite an ambivalent feeling to the father underneath. He was a mischievous boy—he would break things and he feared his father's homecoming when a settling-up was necessary. In summer studying, putting off and putting off—he would lie about his having studied. "Father after us all the time, prodding us." "Nagging a bit"—"Still does it and rouses great opposition in me." "I got my back up." "Father always goes ahead and does the thing he asks us to do—we are so slow and he is so impatient." "Hence we lose interest, he had gone ahead and done it." "If we did it, it would be the wrong way anyway." Rarely tender—passive or distant, rarely demonstrative. "When at boarding school would write me a letter, would send a stamped addressed envelope—as if demanding a reply."

Here one sees outlined much of the hesitancy factors which enter into the patient's business and social difficulties. His reluctance to push himself forward under the father anxiety supervision. His dissociation of anxiety (jumping the gap) and wanting help to get out of straddling the gap, and as I take it the homoerotic fixation—deep underneath father attachment and its ambivalent: *i.e.*, his narcissistic mother identification—(one woman got off on the father floor); also dream of two days later. *Had been playing squash; was coming down elevator with two men. Some sort of entertainment then going on. Two men disappeared leaving me quite alone. I was averse—no drink—diffident. Then a woman got hold of me and took me to a bench, talking to me. She then became a man. I was cornered. The place or recess where we were so low that I could not straighten up. Anxiety and annoyance.*

No new material bearing on the eye situation turned up and I avoided activation as I felt I was treading on rather serious ground as it was. The analysis of the blushing was not without some serious matters for consideration and I was struck with certain resemblances in the dream material with those of a patient seen for a very short time some years previously (1915), whose social inhibitions, general diffused blushing and unconscious homoerotic situation—which at a later time eventuated in suicide while he was under the care of an internist.

Thus a dream of April 8th: *I want to keep an appointment with you at your office which had been changed to the ground floor of a building we manage in East 54th Street. I was accompanied by the business manager, who showed me with great pride a mirror and table he had bought for the hall. This man followed me in your office and sat down. After you had been talking for a short time I decided to get rid of him and excused myself on the ground of having to show him something in the basement. On returning I noticed you had to pass through a bathroom in order to reach your office and you were wearing a pink dressing gown. After we had gotten started you told me that you had found out that you would not be able to help me without fatal results to myself. I replied that if you would not go on with the process I would be dead anyway within a year from alcohol and pleaded with you to take a chance.*

This dream was analyzed only as to some of its more superficial aspects. It with others had given me the impression that Nature might possibly be a better therapist than I and that I might here have an illustration of the principle which strikes me as quite sound, namely that symbolic castration—which appears in the form of organic deformation or malformation or irreversible organic disease process—may be a compromise formation which enables the individual to remain in the herd at the expense of a part of his body (*das Es*).

In saying this I am not unmindful of the very frequent experience which has been frequently commented upon of the capacity during analysis, when a libido-transfer situation is loosened, of the regression to an early instinctive phase in the ontogeny of the individual. How with each new advance in the depths of the psychical systems the regression becomes deeper. With many another I have started with " hysterical " conversion symptoms and apparently arrived at " schizophrenic " levels.[5] Even more pronounced have been the recurrent thoughts in working through the regression scale of organic cases, that one peers into the chasm of a severe catatonic splitting possibility.

Bodily disease may constitute the sacrifice for mental, *i.e.,* herd, conformity—which when failing may permit a severe withdrawal from the herd either by suicide or any of its less radical substitutes.

Thus in the broadest of speculative limning in my first case noted the myopia possibly made a herd adjustment (marriage relation) possible. The wife died from a malignant disease before thirty-three. As hinted, this may be understood some day in terms of unconscious dynamics. The narcissistic fixation of the myopic husband may have denied the woman the baby—hence her organic disease displacement, possibly complicated

[5] See Alexander, F., *loc. cit., Metapsychologische Darstellung*, p. 172. Compare Alexander, F., " Der biologische Sinn psychischer Vorgänge," *Imago*, Bd. IX, 1923.

by her idealistic sexual morality and her own marriage to herself in the terms of her husband's female component.

This break is then followed by extra stress thrown upon the homo-erotic component—he never remarries—remaining true to the image of the dead wife—*ergo*—the mother fixation—and then a secondary bit of organic pathology comes in—since the social adjustment, tact, diplomacy, finesse, bedside manner, etc., etc., are superlative—and a diabetic situation represents an additive *lex talonis* factor—speaking in terms of a definite psychopathology and a questionable absolute ethics.[6]

My information in my second case is fragmentary but here the perverse urge increasingly demanding some form of recognition thrusts more and more energy over to the myopic situation which being insufficient is being balanced by a growing paranoid psychotic behavioristic expression.

In some such manner of thinking are we justified in seeing the myopia-alcohol situation of the patient whose dreams have just been partly pre-sented.   Theoretical considerations would justify a long discussion of their many features, but with these I am not now concerned.   I only think it true that pubertal handling of the narcissistic phase of the Œdipus situation, which stated all too briefly means a specific type of homosexual craving—by an organic castration displacement, which as it were "encysts" libido, constitutes a psychotherapeutic consideration of much moment.   In terms of our quotation from Hawthorne, we cannot deal with the "symptom," *i.e.*, the organic disease as such alone.   Would it not correspond even by the more skillful weapons of the analytic tech-nique, to the cruder stages of hysteria therapy for instance, which deemed it had done something when the symptom was dissipated?   And are not such conversion situations being displaced continuously by innumerable forms of pseudo-therapy?   Symptom analysis is no longer a tenable single goal in the psychoanalysis of the neuroses, or psychoses.[7]

These considerations are advanced relative to the serious underlying libido concealments behind irreversible organic disease, which by locking up libido—a fixed cathexis—acts conversely, for the masses, incapable of greater utilization of the libidinal sources of inspiration.

---

[6] v. Monokow: *The Emotions, Morality and the Brain*, Nervous and Mental Disease Monograph Series, 39. Holt: *The Freudian Wish and Its Relation to Ethics*, 1913.

[7] Rank and Ferenczi: *Development of Psycho-analysis*. Nervous and Mental Disease Monograph Series, 42, 1924.

X.

THE ECOLOGICAL PRINCIPLE IN MEDICINE *

Before I launch into my presentation of the evening I wish to make one comment about a certain setting that I wish to emphasize. It deals more particularly with my use of an unusual term in medicine but one much in vogue in the biological sciences. It is the term ecology—or as we shall see more clearly the large problem of adaptation to physico-chemical, to sensorimotor, and to symbolic or sociogenic forces within the organism and in the environment. Just why I introduce this apparently strange term I hope will become clearer as I proceed.

Ecology is a word that stands for a development of natural history. Certain writers have said it was nothing more than scientific natural history which may be said to have been inaugurated by Buffon in the beginning of the Eighteenth Century, continued by von Humboldt, Malthus, Darwin, Geoffrey, St. Hilaire to Haeckel, who in 1869 first popularized the word Ecology and defined it best, for the purpose to which I would put it, as " the study of the relation of the animal to its organic as well as its inorganic environment, particularly *its friendly or hostile relations* to those animals or plants with which it comes in contact." Haeckel spoke of it as the " general economy of the household of nature." In more modern phraseology, then, the study of " adaptation of man as a whole to the whole of the cosmos."

This is the principle—only fragments of which I can hope to offer for your kindly consideration.

Even the amateur naturalist notes early the numerous devices by which the " struggle for existence " is facilitated and how adaptive activities hint at environmental variations. As a youth tramping over the higher Adirondack metamorphic gneiss rocks, running across a specimen of the rare walking fern—*Camptosorus*—meant that a limestone inclusion must have been found and that further search would reveal certain rarer mosses, hepatics, lichens, ferns, and other plant forms, perhaps in small areas of a dozen yards or so. These were

* Address before the Central Neuropsychiatric Association, Topeka, Kansas, October 25, 1935. Reprinted by permission from *The Journal of Abnormal and Social Psychology,* Vol. 32, No. 1, April-June, 1937.

quite foreign to the plants that grew among the gneisses and granites. Here is an ecological problem of soil adaptation.

Such examples led to thoughts about floras and faunas that were of the woods, and those of the marshes, of the sand dunes, the higher rocky ranges, and many a tramp or ride was spiced with the added enjoyment of reading Nature's methods of adaptation to the environment.

As a student of medicine certain aspects of an analogous nature kept recurring but the subject matter seemed chaotic. There were numerous philosophies of disease. There were obvious adaptations of significance, such as hypertrophies of the heart, of the kidneys, of the muscles, and numerous other organ compensations and correlations with which all of you are familiar.

Should one care to review the cretinoid defects one has the partial problem of habitat with its possible if not probable iodine deficiency factor as determining such a type of development, much as in my illustration of the walking fern, for example. Or, again, many competent studies of dental anomalies seem to show that a disproportionate excess of calcium salts over the organic constituents in teeth development, while possibly making for aesthetic whiteness, on the other hand, favor early decay. If such be the case, then habitat again plays a large part in the admittedly bad teeth of many individuals using water and food products drawn from chalky soils, notably as in certain parts of England and elsewhere.

These, however, are isolated and localized examples of the pertinence of the ecological principle of much less complexity than those to which your attention is directed in this paper.

All these lie on the surface. It is only here and there one catches an inkling of relationships as to such complicated correlations as between old maids and honey of the Darwinian story, for instance. Or the even more complicated correlations of overparasitization of politicians in the social aggregate, widely recognized as the disease of bureaucracy.

I can well remember the thrill concerning the "wisdom of the body," a term much in use by the ancients and recently well elaborated by Cannon, when the possible advantages of fever as a bactericide were first broached by our professor of pathology. No one then had an inkling of the service to which the malarial fever could be brought to serve in the attack upon *Treponema pallida*. The "open issues" of the ancients, yes, even the "tenons" and

" poxes " of the even more ancient Chinese, belong in related categories. I might wander far and wide and gather an enormous mass of quaint and forgotten lore illustrative of these larger problems of what nowadays are mostly dealt with by the immunologist or allergist. But I must narrow myself down to a much more limited horizon.

It is within my own lifetime that a large group of disorders satirized by Molière as " les maladies imaginaires," termed the " vapors " and hypochondriacal disorders by the English, Cheyne and others, have swung into line as illustrations of the principle of adaptation and of compromise, in the understanding of which the ecological principle of the ideologcal environment plays so important a rôle.

In looking about for an entry into the confines of a large group of organismic reactions which for centuries have been called the " mimics," or the shadows of disease, and which I may use to illustrate one of the issues of the optimistic biological aspect of compensatory adaptation, I have gone back to the Greeks and first to Democritus.

We are not concerned here with his atomic theory generalization, important as it has been, but more particularly with his explanation of a type of behavior disorder which even in his day evidently was not uncommon. You all know that Hippocrates took over more or less an idea from Democritus, clothing the conception in such terms as the " moving uterus," which gave rise to difficulties in numerous parts of the body, one of the most striking of which at that time was termed the " globus hystericus."

Here were the beginnings of a study of a process of adaptation which has come to be more carefully investigated in recent times under the conception of conversion and organ libido investment.

Democritus was no fool, nor Hippocrates neither. I do not believe that either of them was so crude or anatomically so poorly oriented as to believe that the actual organ, the uterus, wandered about the body, when, as in " globus hystericus," it lodged in the throat seeking for impregnation.

I am persuaded that Democritus was speaking of the instinct for reproduction which might seize upon every organ of the body to attempt to express itself symbolically. Thus I am certain that in his time there were others than the Thracians who believed in the principle of the " body as a whole " as Socrates has so clearly elaborated in Plato's Charmides and to which I shall return, I hope, with something other than merely lip service. Thus I am again persuaded that Democritus realized that there were affections of the body which were of idealistic construction. His hysteria stands out as a striking example, and the mechanisms of displacement and of conversion, as we now speak of them, had been observed and described and even more, partly interpreted, much as in the present day mode. It goes without saying, however, lacking the clinching proof of the detailed unfolding as well as the dynamic economic utility of symptom formation which the study of the Unconscious has revealed since the advent of Freud.

So as I read Galen's somewhat pretentious argumentation as to the foolishness of the conception of Democritus, I think we should realize that Galen here showed a lack of that " temperance of judgment " which was so highly thought of and spoken of among the thinkers of Greece. His demonstration of the broad ligaments as preventing any such wandering uterus and his Q.E.D., as to the occurrence of the hysterical disorder in men, without any uterus, reminds me of much self-satisfied assertion concerning many " opinions," these and those, where the " all or none " principle is invoked. Either good or bad, black or white, God or the Devil, sane or insane, body or mind, mental or physical, these have been the naïve realistic bulwarks of nominalistic argumentation through all times, forgetful of Zeno's celebrated arrow that did not move because of this " all or nothing " type of anal sadistic desire for the " infallible."

To the Greeks, of the times of which I speak, temperance meant " wisdom." A wisdom which expressed itself in their search for a better adaptation to the laws of the gods—*i.e.,* of the natural forces that they were so curious about with the effort at mastering. Plato's dialogue entitled Charmides—perhaps an old story to most of you— dealt with Temperance in just this aspect. A temperance not of purely oral drinking and eating pleasures, but that steady self-control in the indulgence of all the feelings and habits which a sensible education was held to be its object. This is the temperance that Socrates identified with wisdom. Xenophen [1] pointed this out early and down through the ages many have followed this interpretation. The " Synthesis of the Ego " is one of its present day facets expressed in the psychoanalytic terminology.

Inasmuch as the " Charmides " [2] opens on a note of definitely

[1] Xenophen, M. S., III, 9, 4.
[2] Chiefly from Burges translation. Bohn Library Edition. Vol. IV. London: George Bell & Sons, 1906.

medical tone, permit me to repeat a bit of the theme. Socrates has just returned from one of the wars of the day and desirous of learning what was doing respecting philosophy and respecting the young men, whether they had been remarkable for wisdom or beauty or both, was introduced to Charmides, "who is thought to be the most beautiful of all at the present time." Socrates falls in with the universal admiration but first asks Critias, the tutor of Charmides, "If in his soul should he be so well formed?" And so the introduction takes place under the old familiar ruse of bringing him in contact with a physician touching a weakness lately spoken of, namely, a "heaviness in the head when he awakens in the morning."

Charmides soon asks Socrates if he knew the remedy, and—I ask you to take note, Socrates replying yes—states, "It is a certain *leaf*," "and a certain *incantation* in addition to the medicine." Both must be used. And the incantation? asks Charmides, and the answer! "For this incantation is such, that it is able to make the head sound; but, as perhaps you have learned from clever physicians, when anyone comes to them with a pain in their eyes, who say that they must not attempt to cure the eyes alone, but that it is necessary for them at the same time to attend to the head, if the eyes are to be in a good state, or on the other hand, that it would be great stupidity to think of attending to the head alone without the whole body." "In consequence of this very reasoning, they turn themselves to the whole body, and by diet (and regimen) endeavor to attend to and cure the part together with the whole."

Then, [and you will pardon me if I bring corn to Kansas] Socrates goes on to say that he had learned this from one of the Thracian physicians who first credits the thesis to the Greeks but goes on to boast a bit, saying that their king, being a god, says it is not proper to attempt to cure the eyes without the head nor the head without the body, so neither is it proper to cure the body without the soul, and this was the reason why many disease escape the Greek physicians—note the eternal chauvinistic tendency—because they are ignorant of the whole." "For all things proceed from the soul, both the good and the bad, to the body and to the whole man"—and further "that the soul was cured by certain incantations; and that these incantations were *beautiful reasons;* and that such temperance was generated in the soul, which when generated and present can easily impart health both to the head and to the rest of the body." "Let none," says Socrates, "persuade you to cure his head with this medicine (the certain leaf) who shall not have first presented his soul to be cured by you with the incantation. For the fault of the present time respecting men is this (how modern the note) that certain persons endeavor to become physicians without a knowledge of either (temperance or health)."

As I turn the pages of many a volume on the history of medicine I am amazed at finding this same story interpreted in a manner which, to me, seems strangely at variance with its import. In these histories incantations are spoken of as exorcisms, as charms, and the whole congeries of wish-fulfilling devices. Socrates, you note, defined incantations as "*beautiful reasons*" and we know that to the Greeks beautiful meant "*true.*" Their chief concern was this search for the beautiful—*i.e.,* the essence of *truth*—in everything, and we know to what heights and depths they attained in their sculpture, their architecture, their drama—which existing today in fixed forms, are accurate indications of the achievements they must have reached in all other human activities.

The study of "disease," using this word in its largest meaning, may be said to be a branch of Ecology. Ecology, or in the sense here taken, scientific natural history, is a relatively modern term. I shall not burden this paper further with the story of its historical develop- ment.[3] Etymologically it means the study of "*home relations*" of organisms; for our purpose, then, the study of environmental adap- tation of organisms—whole—and in the medical phase a study of ecological factors of maladaptation of organisms as a whole—in the true Socratic sense already outlined. It is further defined as a "science of communities." If thus rigorously delimited my intended use of certain concepts of ecology are somewhat distorted—for cer- tain ecologists have claimed that a study of the relations of a single species (and much more a certain individual of the species) to the environment conceived without reference to communities and in the end, unrelated to the natural phenomena of its habitat and com- munity associates, is not properly included in the field of ecology. No such individual can exist apart from its community, nor unre- lated to the natural phenomena of its habitat and community asso- ciates, hence the accent here on the ecological conception of "adap- tation and particularly maladaptation *as a whole to the whole.* Surely a program large enough to inhibit any mortal. Inasmuch as I shall not offer you the whole pie but only a small bite of it, I can perhaps

[3] Consult Chapman, R. N., Animal Ecology, for this and other pertinent material. New York: McGraw-Hill Book Co., 1931.

do no better than to cut off a small wedge by offering my own " heaviness in the head " to psychopathophysiological scrutiny. Perhaps I shall succeed only in offering a bit of biotic ecological pastry with a seedy raisin or two.

There are those, and perhaps they are in the majority, whose thoughts, concerning certain issues I would raise, go somewhat as follows: It has been said that ecology, when reduced to its lowest terms by a process of analysis, becomes physiology; that physiology when similarly reduced becomes a physiological chemistry; that physiological chemistry may be resolved to biochemistry, it in its turn to pure chemistry, and finally to physical chemistry until we touch bottom in physics and mathematics. For some this is the only scientific program, difficult as it may be to reduce a maladaptive medical situation to such fundamentals. Kraus, in his Clinical Synthesis (Sysziologie), I take it, approaches medical problems from this side.

Let me present a bit of myself from a variant point of view.[4] It is now some few years since I have noted, what rarely happened before, that when a door suddenly slams, or the telephone rings, I suddenly start. Again at times more particularly after a long day's work, or on a day following broken sleep, if perchance someone brushes by my foot or leg, an instantaneous tetaniform kick is set off in my touched extremity. Later and even more annoyingly I catch myself just in time as I partly turn my head around to see something moving behind me, just realizing that it is but a glint from behind of something seen at the edge of my glasses.

Hearing, touching, seeing perceptions are mentioned; all quite different as to their anatomical pathways, and their sensory fields, yet allied somewhere, I am certain, in the sphere of interpretation and of causality. In short, I am " jumpy." Possibly a Chvostek or Trousseau sign might have been demonstrated and other " spasmophilic " signs if tested by chronaxia.

A few more bits of evidence should be added to my indictment. Not infrequently I find myself turning suddenly to the right— strangely never to the left—at some moving body. This time the faulty perception is not from my glasses but from a prominent hair of my eyebrow, or a hanging object like a lamp bulb that comes between me and a window and for the moment creates the illusion of

[4] Already touched upon in paper by Jelliffe, " Acroparesthesia and Quinidine, A Quest and a Query." *J. Nerv. and Ment. Dis.*, 79: 631, 1934.

a passing stranger. Then again in my room, shared by my secretary and part of my library, I have a double row of cabinets, each drawer one above the other with its small white label into which reprints are sorted according to their respective groupings—à la Jelliffe and White. Time and time again, as I have passed through this room to my consulting room, and again on the right, I compulsively turn to give a quick glance at this set-up because of a provoking, semi-hallucinatory identification of a bellboy in smart uniform or a Park avenue doorman or some such military figure.

We are here encroaching on an interesting physiological field which you will recall Henry Head entitled " Vigilance " and which, in the instances recited, passes over the pathophysiological border to a hypervigilance. Fortunately—I at least assume—at the border that protects the Ego there is sufficient anticathexis, and a prompt correction of the illusory images, in the visual field at least, which prevents the breaking through of the Id for hallucinatory formation, and the reality function of the Ego stands up in spite of some trouble somewhere on the line from receptor periphery to center and/or in the reverse effector direction.

What, however, has produced this hypervigilance which reveals itself as a kick, a start, a turn of the head, and what relationship has it to the " economy of the household "?

The spasmophilic type of motility, as a specimen, is clearly comparable to my finding of the walking fern, and, an ecological factor, calcium, coincidentally, is implicated. In terms of emergent levels [5] in the body from Matter (chemistry—calcium), to Life (biology—motor response), to Mind (psychology—illusory—hallucinatory images)—there is no doubt about them all being involved—and that if ecology be reduced to biochemistry then the calcium alteration in the environment, *i.e.*, the ionic milieu, is the main culprit.

When this exposé of my " innards " was first made, I was content to speak of a spasmophilia and a probable calcium deficiency. The outgo was greater than the income. The blood chemistry, however, showed that the ionic milieu was kept up by some masterly homeo-kinesis—the household economy was regulated in some way. Maybe Peter was robbing to pay Paul. And so I found it to be, for, happening for other reasons to have an X-ray status of my joints taken, I learned that my skull bones had been worked for calcium to such an extent that I had a Paget skull. It had been literally riddled by

[5] Smuts, Holism, 1933.

pickpockets. Even before this type of inner household compensatory borrowing was discovered the well known lessons from hyperventilation were called to mind. Hyperventilation as is well known tends to exhaust CO_2 held in the alveoli, which in its turn disturbs the acid-base equilibrium. In order to make good, Ca, or other bivalent kations, are called upon as the alkali reserve is depleted. Breathing habits offered some speculative issues and the forms of breathing as seen in catatonic precox cases and in encephalitic cases were reviewed.

Finally I looked at some of my own motor habits in breathing, and, here I ask your special attention, since possibly an insight might be gained as to very definite factors of ecological significance.

For years I have been aware of a certain compulsion-repetition type of breathing, especially when talking. As I am somewhat of a stranger to most of you, in this connection, I would say that the habit consisted largely in the drive to get the largest number of words out of every breath I exhale. I squeeze out words to the bitter end before I take my next breath. Thus unwittingly, and even when I became aware of the practice, I have been hyperventilating all of the time I talk. Inasmuch as at times I talk too much, it is not difficult to perceive how I have been robbing one part of my body, calling on other parts to maintain the budget. Were I not ambivalently mute for long periods, I had been gathered to my fathers long ere this.

Just what has happened to my parathyroids in these onslaughts on my calcium I am not aware of, nor am I certain that the parathyroids alone are the only sufferers. Whether reversible functional adenomatous parathyroid tissues are there, or suprarenal correlations are also present, I suspect some alliance, because of a related ready fatigability which is also handled much like the breathing.

This is not all, for I am convinced that other expressor functions operate along related lines. In my writing the sentence formation tends in the same direction. If I am not careful my sentences are of the German type wherein clause after clause is strung together with the verbal close some pages from the beginning. This, I suspect, has been going on for many years. Like the breathing, I seem to wish to get it all down in one large philosophical whole. As a matter of history I can recall a comment once made by my brother who, listening to me talk when a young man, said that he often held his breath wondering if I would come out right in my sentence before I got through. I shall spare you other revelations concerning methods of work, tendencies to collect huge masses of material; desires to leave no stone of historical moment unturned. My bibliographies have a tendency to swamp my production. By the time I have amassed a mountain of information, my little mouse of an individual contribution is lost in the mountain.

The psychoanalytically alert listener can put his finger on an aspect of the trouble in an instant. The breathing and all of the other related effector responses are following an infantile oral-anal patterning. As in childhood, I am repeating the " try hard " formula so well known in the privy chamber—realistically as well as symbolically.

The kernel of my discussion is thus revealed. The psychoanalyst thinks of the displacement mechanisms as well as the compulsive substitutions.

The biochemical alteration is undoubtedly there. The altered chemism is unquestionably correlated with the hypervigilance phenomena of the semi-hallucinatory experiences. I am further inclined to give credence to the thought that were I not a bit deaf auditory illusions might come alongside of the optical and motor ones. I might even go still further and argue that in conformity with the compensatory efforts of my household economy that the deafness itself may have arisen as a protective device against such falsifications of reality.

I am assuming that the Ego function of repression, coupled with tyrannical Super-Ego cathectic coöperation, has aided in the prevention of falsifications in the optic sphere and psychotic interpretations have been held back.

The real difficulty lies not primarily in the altered chemism but in the oral-anal libidinous cathexis which would strive for oratorical, rhetorical supremacy. To complete the Œdipus formula I might add that such a drive is undoubtedly a remnant of an identification with a striving to surpass my father. He, among other things, was a trained elocutionist. I never became one.

I have given a thumb-nail sketch—albeit a large and sore thumb— of what a following out of the ecological principle demands should we as neuropsychiatrists wish to understand disease processes, other than those in which the Ego repression barrier is more or less easily or periodically broken through, notably as in certain psychoses and in certain phases of the psychoneuroses.

The ecological principle demands information of a total quality.

It is not satisfied at a chemical explanation alone, nor one at the biological level alone, nor yet one at the purely psychological level— all three must give of their fraction in the total picture. Just what the intricate equating at these roughly indicated levels may be, constitutes the work of the conscientious neo-Hippocratic physician.

And now I would turn to certain of the definite issues that make up certain of the problems which the neuropsychiatrist must some day solve. I am persuaded that the internists of the present modes cannot do so, since in the last analysis they are not equipped to master the phenomena and even more the dynamic situations at the psychological, or if you prefer the sociogenic level. It is here that man as a social animal must put forth his most strenuous efforts at adaptation.

The precursors of human bioplasm have had billions of years of experience at the chemical level. His animal ancestors have struggled for millions of years with various physiological adaptive compromises.

Were it not for the " vis medicatrix naturae," which is but a latinically expressed intuition of these truths, where would the doctor of today be in his handling of the great run of human discomforts? Whereas automatic adjustments have had these long time binding experiences, it has been only within the comparatively short span of some hundred thousand years or even fewer that man has had to deal with more explicitly condensed group ideologies as environmental realities. I shall not expand the picture but would make but one comment, that whereas the " wisdom of the body " may serve now an excellent summary of his internal adaptive mechanisms, Socrates' " incantations " for the soul as " beautiful reasons " may be invoked equally as a guide for his ideological adaptations.

Our formula then takes on this peculiar possibility—that, apart from accident, much chronic so-called organic disease is a type of conservative response to such ideological adaptations. In order to stay in the herd, i.e., not become psychotic, and be turned out to grass as the Nebuchadnezzar prototype, one of the modes of compromise adaptation has been some form of somatic destruction, reversible or irreversible. The figure of speech of " flight into an illness " is more than a fiction. It is a bit of stark reality, but more on the heroic side of the scale are those whose resistances are such that, like the classical Spartan youth, they allow the fox of displaced libido to gnaw and ultimately to consume their vitals.

However, as is manifest not in medicine alone but in all scientific fields, theoretical, interpretative formulations are far ahead of the ability to apply them to all concrete situations.

Thus, as in geophysics, a great deal is known about earthquakes. They can be predicted and located with a fair degree of accuracy, still no one as yet, through such knowledge, has shooed off an earthquake.

In a handful of sand, we learn from the physical chemists, there is an enormous amount of heat locked up, but no one yet has been able to fry an egg with a pebble.

I do not know whether we shall do our cooking with sand before or after we have solved the problem of the application of the principles which I have briefly touched upon for the unraveling of innumerable situations in clinical medicine. I do feel that we have made a beginning in the last 30–40 years in this latter field and this has come chiefly through the work of Freud on the dynamic conceptions of the *libido* and the field of the *unconscious*.

The great run of human beings refuse to alter their repetition compulsions, *i.e.,* their habits. These represent their infantile pleasure principle patterns, and when such meet with reality they compromise in some form of illness from which they resist being torn loose. The dynamic principles involved in organic distortions, which almost invariably begin most insidiously as neurotic disturbances are slowly being understood. Much of this has been intuitively grasped since earliest time. Even the latest " Handbuch der Neurologie " speaks of the " *so-called* organ neuroses." While in this stage of distortion or compensation the physiological processes and colloidal structure changes are still reversible. Every one and sometimes nearly all of the organs of the body from the skin outside to the blood inside show these efforts at ecological adaptation to faulty patterns of action. There is an ancient saw that speaks of a " doctor or a fool at forty." In this, our present setting, we may interpret this as meaning that if by forty one has not become really creative he develops an organic irreversible process out of what was once a reversible process. Expressed in another way, " *Behavior pattern has eaten its way into anatomical pattern and will not be recalled.*"

Just where to begin in any review of these irreversible, *i.e.,* malignant or chronic organic conversion patterns, is not easy to decide. Logically speaking, the skin would seem to come first, but I shall start with the organs of movement. The earliest known animals, the

Amoeba, has locomotive organs which it can produce in accordance with the situation.

In Jelliffe and White (Ed. VI, p. 245) the conception of the muscle-joint-bone trilogy as forming an early unit to meet gravitational and inertia stimuli is elaborated. Of the many situations which develop from frustrations and which utilize this trilogy I shall point to but one, *i.e.,* the arthritis problem.

In the long history of medicine, disorders of the muscle, tendon, joint apparatus stand out again as evidence of our lack of adequate understanding. In spite of magnificent advances made here as in all fields of medicine, some chronic arthritides remain hard nuts to crack. Recent trends have segregated two large " niches "—termed respectively " rheumatoid arthritis," in which infectious parasites seem to play a predominant rôle, and " osteoarthritis," seemingly of different etiology and reflecting metabolic factors independent of infection.

Our program would deal with the infectious types as with other parasitic adaptations. Here problems of habitat are of significance. What of the soil that permits the invasion? Why is it that but about 1 to 2 per cent of the population have rheumatoid arthritis and yet 100 per cent of us harbor the specific parasitic enemies in our intestines, teeth, sinuses, tonsils, etc., All honor to bacteriological and immunological research and more of it, but the deep unconscious factors of the personality of the individuals infected should not be left uninvestigated.

As for many of the osteoarthritides, however, there are some very pertinent studies to be made relative to the unconscious muscular tensions of love and of hate, of impatience and of haste, of grasping and of greed, of hauling and pulling, of aggressive hostile striking, beating, and a host of other maladaptive tensions which express themselves in the muscle-tendon-joint trilogy.[6] There is no doubt in the mind of the neuropsychiatrist that maladaptive tensions in these structures can and do modify the metabolism of the joints. They tend in no small measure to bring about changes which lock up the points in arthritic bondage after months or years of faulty tensions.

The antisocial individual whose repressive and suppressive unconscious and/or conscious mechanisms are unable to check his hostile

---

[6] See Jelliffe and White, " Diseases of Nervous System," Ed. VI, 1935, pp. 245 *et seq.* Lea & Febiger, Philadelphia.

aggressive impulses gets locked up in jail. The irony of the wheel chair waits for the like individual who, finding no better way to pull the world to pieces, or to batter it into compliance with his wishes, and yet would stay in the herd, essentially and intrincisally unproductive in some part of his personality, punishes himself and by the ecologically determined osteoarthritic device.

Permit me a short description of one of many an illustrative example. Some more drastic and tragic situations are in my case records. Discretion prevents the portrayal of some of the most striking. A fifty-year-old man whom I had known socially since boyhood hobbled into my office all tied up. He was down and out and sympathy was the only coin in the picture. X-ray studies, gratuitously provided by a competent and high minded colleague, revealed a widespread crippling osteoarthritis.

To those interested in " so-called " heredity, it appears his father was a bit gouty; his mother was an osteoarthritic at eighty and a sister ten years older than he was markedly involved in a similar type of osteoarthritis, albeit both mother and sister were " nice " people. There were three in the family at the time of his birth; a ten year older sister and a fourteen month older brother with whom it would appear there was an intense though not open rivalry. When he was born the older brother was taken care of by the sister. He became mother's special pride, joy and disappointment more openly than was the older brother. In fact he was very chummy with his mother even to adult years.

He was smarter, socially, than the older brother, although intellectually the senior was in the lead. They were both typical boys who grew up together on the outskirts of a large city, were on the same baseball teams, football teams, etc. The younger brother was very keen of eye and gathered in all the marbles and tops of the neighborhood. The older brother was a plodder; usually did his lessons first and then was ready to play, the younger played first and worked after. Neither one nor the other were ever " left back " but the younger was impatient, wanted to get ahead, make money and went to a commercial school, while the older plugged away at a profession, which delayed his marriage until nearly thirty, while the younger one married earlier and once remarked to his sister-in-law, " I got ahead of him there ! " He was a successful salesman and proprietor but a spendthrift and happy-go-lucky, a fisherman and card player, not a gambler. There were children; divorce, remarriage, and finally widowed about fifty he lived with two daughters, one having been married and had had a daughter.

His elder daughter was trying to get a divorce and I saw him in the midst or towards the end of this legal entanglement.

The father-daughter fixations were obvious on the surface and in his story as he poured it out to me. For some two or three years before he came to see me he was all tied up in a snarl of economic and emotional conflicts revolving about the divorce. His hatred of the son-in-law was such that only " liquidation," in the U. S. S. R. sense, would have satisfied it. As he sat in my office, in the full light of the usual physician's window or paced the floor, he ranted the prolonged, tedious, and harassing story of the trials, counter trials, etc., etc. As he did so his face and bodily musculature were all twisted into the form he would that his opponents might be reduced to. His knitted and gnarled fingers comported them-selves as tearing tools of torture for the son-in-law, judges, lawyers, and all the adversaries. The mildest form of action that his whole motor attitude, including his speech, would indicate was to " rip out their guts." He was beaten at every turn of the procceeding and I saw him when the thing was boiling over.

Fortunately he was not altogether dumb psychologically and once put on the track of what these hostile, aggressive, and sadistic drives were doing to his muscular tensions and thus to the joints, he learned the harm-fulness of such attitudes. His violent and prolonged rages, he came to realize, were only putting him further and further into a wheel chair as a helpess cripple.

I have had the opportunity to get much insight into the unconscious of a few wheel chair osteoarthritic individuals. Doré's famous pictures of a burning hell might well describe these glimpses. On the outside veneer they were all as sweet as honey or as placid as a mill pond.

My patient's interior was probably a roaring furnace judged by the sparks and heat of his motor tensions. He, as stated, took a tumble to himself and mended his ways so that he made some very substantial recovery. His economic situation was far from satisfactory. A small fortune had gone out in the legal conflict. A sublime faith in the success of his future possibilities—a million just around the corner—was one of his supporting and helpful consolations. An ever optimistic personality had been encouraged to the limit almost of delusional belief. The grasp-ing at the future finally took more and more of his sadistic-hostile muscle joint aims and thus these mechanisms were able to function more successfully.

Anything like an analysis was precluded. I could promise him nothing more than a purely academic survey of unconscious func-tioning. However, what little I did offer gave much better returns than had the tooth pulling, diathermy, uterus, ovarian curetting, hormone therapy, etc., etc., that had been carried out for the sister and mother for twenty years or more. I have known the family sixty years.

While from the beginning the human organism feels with his periphery, and hence my temptation to start with the skin, we undoubtedly move in response to gravitational stimuli before birth. The foetus unquestionably smells, hears, and possibly distinguishes light. Of the myelinated tracts, Flechsig showed early the signifi-cance of those connected with equilibration and movement begins about the fifth month. But he breathes only after birth. The lungs come into operation only at that time.

I shall limit my remarks here, other than those already mentioned as to certain breathing habits, chiefly to the subject of tuberculosis, one of the outstanding challenges to medicine. The tubercle bacillus, even though necessary, is but one of the factors in this war of mycotic parasitism. Every man harbors the tubercle bacillus. The parasite is universal. Only a few of us succumb to the fungus. The ecological principle demands more information concerning the soil that permits the parasite to use it as a medium for its persistence, and in my opinion it is not irrelevant to emphasize that may be the personality of the lung is of more importance to study than the bio-chemical life of the fungus parasite.

Here the modern psychiatric methodology has but few systema-tized observations to offer in spite of the colossal mass of information about the struggle of adaptation, i.e., the disease. It has found, however, in these few studies the preponderating influence of the Death Wish. The flight into the tuberculous disease has been found to be a regressive return to the Nirvana of intrauterine happiness in its extremist forms and in the stopping at many way stations on the regressive pathway. For some it is the sadomasochistic expression of " You'll be sorry when I'm gone," so familiar to wounded nar-cissism. " Who will deny me the pleasure of seeing a world mourn at my loss? ", some may recall as the cry of the suiciding hero in a comparatively recent drama—and the philosopher's acid and stringent reply, " The world, my boy, will say, one less mouth to feed." How true to the ecological principle of ultimate food survival values!

Again other tuberculous individuals show their unconscious " revenge " motive which has grown up from infantile rivalries and interpretations of fancied favors to sister or brother or to other specially hostile elements. Here the same motivating projection and introjection mechanisms are revealed as heavily cathected as made familiar in the suicidal drives of the depressed manic. Here the " partial " or " organ " suicide motive is paramount.[7]

The gradations of the " prostitution complex " in the tuberculous are innumerable.

Just as man does not live to eat alone, so he does not use his lungs only for purposes of oxygen-carbon dioxide relationship. He uses

---

[7] Menninger, K.: " Focal Self Destruction," *Am. Jour. Psychiat.* Jelliffe, S. E.: " What Price Healing," *Jour. Am. Med. Assoc.*, 94: 1393, 1930.

his lungs for other purposes. For aspiration as well as for respiration. As a medium of social contact through rich verbalization the lung function is the chief agent through which man's sublimations may keep him effectually healthy.

Is it to be wondered at, then, that a universally distributed parasite should find an ecologically adapted habitat in those organs which, on the principles of unconscious motivation, are failing to come up to complete adult socialized value? I should like to linger with the history of such sadistic individuals as Calvin and Swift and a host of others to demonstrate the thesis further.

Let us go back to the skin. From the days of the Protozoa the outside surface has been exposed to a variety of pressure stimuli, molar as well as molecular. It has been bathed a billion years in ancestral isotonic fluids. In the human womb and later the skin recapitulates these time-bound ecological experiences.

Of the innumerable maladaptive variations I shall touch only on eczema and psoriasis, since these still proffer the raspberry to dermatological interpretation and resist therapeutic efforts.

Is it of significance, the ecological principle demands, that the one should involve preëminently flexor surfaces and exhibit wet or exudative features, whereas the other chiefly involves extensor surfaces and shows preëminently dry scaly characters? As I scan current dermatological literature these aspects of these two outstanding rebels to therapy are not even dreamed of. That skin physicochemical memories must be engraved in their structural integration is undoubted. The skin, as having a mnemic inheritance in its struggles to survive as an efficient ecologically adaptive organ—this notion seems foreign to dermatology, which also may be said to have its pre-Freudian historical period. Even allergic ecphorias may be approached from this point of view.

To those who think with the entire ecological principle and for whom the psychoanalytic methodology is applicable, flexor surfaces have a different significance than extensor ones, just as flexor muscles do different things than extensor ones. The former skin goals are chiefly caressing goals, the latter chiefly rebuffing. On the flexor side of the skin as for muscles there is chiefly grasping, taking, possessing, holding. On the extensor side there is predominantly refusing, rejecting. Thus in eczema and in psoriasis the unconscious psychological fraction of the ecological principle asks how the skin libido operates to activate ambivalent efforts at gratification both in terms of location and in the wet and dry phenomena. How through autopunition (masochistic) and hostile (sadistic) repressed material regressive satisfaction is obtained at secondary and primary narcissistic levels?

Further, the ecological aspect of adaptation queries, why the repulsive acnes of many young adolescents? The gonadal hormones, like the calcium of my kick, etc., unquestionably are involved; but is this all? On the contrary, the methodology that is interested in unconscious motivation reveals other factors, such as the sado-masochistic activities just spoken of. Many such individuals on analysis are found to be punishing their faces to scourge their souls. They put on as repulsive a mask as do the fantastic primitives in their dance ceremonials to frighten away devils, thus displaying their hostility to a world interpreted as hostile, in much the same sense as the masked devil chasers.

Had we the time I could cite at length cases which show how craved and frustrated caressing has been the immediate precursor of mild or even very severe eczematous manifestations. Likewise the significance of hostile sadistic activities in the production of periodic and persistent psoriasis.

I shall mention only one patient—also dealt with elsewhere [8]—with a universal psoriasis which early impressed me and has served as a paradigm, by reason of its malignancy, for a host of minor examples of the same ecological principle. Here was an ambitious, greedy and sadistic personality with a pronounced unconscious criminal drive. This latter was largely held in check by the study of law which bolstered up the Ego defense system. The practice of criminal law was necessary however as both an outlet and as a defense.

There was further extension into economic schemes of social aid to similarly distorted patterns. I refrain, from motives of discretion, from specifying the exact nature of these enterprises, covertly semi-legitimized by current financial, social, and legal "ethics."

During a fragmentary analysis, for other than the skin manifestations particularly, and twenty-five years ago, I asked him, as a plain masochistic dream-expressed drive was evident, " Why do you strive to get in jail? " I would add expressly that the psoriasis symbolically represented, at that time, the equivalent of an intrauterine jail.

In spite of all of the currents and counter currents, the sublimations and repressions, he finally landed in jail. It took twenty-five years or more to achieve the unconscious craving. It is too long a story to detail here.

---

[8] Jelliffe, S. E.: " Organic Disease and Psychopathology." *Am. J. Psychiat.,* 92: 1051, March, 1936.

Of all of the internal organs biology leads us to think of the *heart* as starting early. Even with the early pulsating vacuole of lower forms outside stimuli can affect the beat. The popular and at the same time correct tradition is that many cardiac disturbances are "nervous." This word "nervous," like "emotion," is an omnibus word that means everything and nothing. In the strict neuropsychiatric sense "nervous" really means of mental or "psychogenic"— or "total reaction" origin or participation. Without some tie-up with the Œdipus behavior patterning these words are without much more than descriptive significance. They have little meaning. Conversions, projections, introjections, displacements, these and other mental mechanisms, must be seen in order that a dynamic understanding of the "nervous" or "emotional" symptoms may be obtained. Just as the average neuropsychiatrist is dumb in the reading of an electrocardiogram, so is the average internist as much in a fog concerning the psychoanalytic complexities of the "emotions."[9]

A tachycardiac compulsion neurosis (phobic) response is quite a different thing from a tachycardiac conversion mechanism. It is much more intricate, harder to disentangle, and more questionable as to prognosis and therapy. A projection tachycardia, which is chiefly founded on unconscious homoerotic impulses, is still another kettle of fish. These and a dozen more tachycardias of predominantly psychogenic causation are often helped, even permanently relieved, by an enlightened psychotherapy. The difficult phobic and projection situations usually require psychoanalysis. Milder disorders may be allayed by persuasion. No one doubts the value of the "certain leaf" of the Socratic version, whether digitalis, quinidine, morphine, rest, or diet, but the "incantation" of "truth" is the only remedy for certain of these "emotional" cardiac disturbances.

In the sphere of the vascular tension states the benefits derived from a psychoanalytic therapy have amply demonstrated the ecological principle of faulty adaptations to the ideological environment. Was it not John Hunter who exclaimed that "his very life was in the hands of any wretch who would anger him"? And did not John Hunter actually die of a coronary spasm or thrombosis attack in the midst of an angry debate in a medical society?

Among the prophylactic measures in our textbooks, we read relative to cerebral hemorrhage is the avoidance of straining at stool. Straining at rage may be infinitely worse than straining at stool.

[9] See K. Menninger and C. F. Menninger. *Am. Heart Jour.*, 11:10, 1936.

What lay behind the ancient saw, " Let not the sun go down upon thy wrath," if not some such recognition of the devastating effects of the " passions " upon our body?

As I look about me and see the countless figures on blood pressures, and other accurate and valuable methods of quantitative analysis, I find excellent criteria for gauging " *motion*," *but nothing relative to* " *motive*." I see the façade of urbanity too often a disguise, a thin veneer for intense and strongly invested hostile cravings. " Nice people," " silk gloves," in manner and dress often are but masks for very sadistic personalities. It is no wonder one finds high blood pressures and kidney casts in the urine of many perfect " ladies " and " gentlemen."

Every naturalist has much to say about the sense of smell in the lower animals. The biogenetic principle teaches us that man has all of these attributes, even if repressed in most individuals. Chemical memories, however, are there and in a sense far superior to those of the earlier human and animal forms, in spite of current misconceptions.[10] No animal other than man, when he practices his sense of smell, is as efficient. I know of no other animal who can spot a wine or a cigar with the accuracy of a wine taster (smeller) or cigar expert. Here is an enormous field for investigation, especially dealing with the identifications of body odors of self and of childhood surrounding objects, with their libidinal fixations, repressions, and later regressive possibilities. Here are pertinent problems which involve the common cold, snotty noses, " halitosis," so dear to the advertising pages of our pulps, sinus disease—so frequent among the grasping money searchers, and holders, the constipated and conservative, epileptic seizures (see Dostoiewsky and Flaubert), and a host of related erotic reactions. A complete exposé of these would well rival the tales patterned after the memorable excursions of Marco Polo.

Should I be inclined to be more structurally minded and offer you an analysis of the anatomical pathways from the olfactory receptors, to the corpora mamillaria, tuber cinerea, and hypothalamic nuclei, much profitable information could be offered concerning neuroendocrine behavior—pattern correlations. If, further, the cortical associations into the final receptor fields should call for comment, the pathological pictures in the cornu Ammonis, first revealed by

[10] See Jelliffe and White: " Diseases of Nervous System." Lea & Febiger, Philadelphia. Ed. I, 1915, to VI, 1935. (Olfactory.)

Alzheimer for epileptoid and related manifestations, might offer profitable material for consideration, factual as well as speculative.

After the cry, the "holler," comes the "swaller." Guided chiefly by smell in the beginning, sucking begins, and from mouth to anus the digestive tract begins to function, ecologically; *i.e.,* chemically, physiologically, and psychologically.

It is not a mere dogma to state that as a child sucks at its mother's breast so will it treat the world as an object of attainment throughout life. The reflections of conflict in gastroenterology carry on the traditions. It is, next to the "cry," the breathing symbol-making organ, the one to which retreat is made in response to frustration. The illnesses, major or minor, that come later reflect in no uncertain manner the early tendencies of the nursing infant.

Regurgitation, greediness, impulsiveness, constipations, diarrheas, indigestions, dyspepsias, ulcers, appendicitis, diverticulitis, gall stones, yes, maybe even carcinomata, are conditioned by personality mal-adaptations displaced to the gastrointestinal functions and structures.

These disorders, may I emphasize, like others referred to, I would state again are not to be considered solely in the light of faulty libidinal distribution. That is, the psychological component is not necessarily the only factor, but every day horse-sense shows us how often this factor is involved and in large amounts. A proper evaluation, in coöperation with biochemical or physiological measuring techniques of *what part* and *how much* unconscious forces are operating is imperative if one aspires to be a good gastroenterologist or even an ordinary doctor.

Lest the inclusion of carcinoma in my list seem extreme, let me add that as yet the factors are too deeply hidden to permit more than suggestive lines of research, but I do stand on the platform that the ignoring of psychological methods as parts of the program of research for the ultimate understanding of carcinomatous or other malignant processes is stupid beyond any understanding.

Thus might I turn our inadequate beam of understanding on unconscious forces as they operate on all of the organs of the body. These organs are bits of structuralized experience—they are somatic precipitates of functioning cravings. Not one of them, maybe not even an isolated blood cell—to go the limit—can act absolutely alone. The billion-year time-bound contacts with the cosmos have forced an integration far beyond any present day intelligence to adequately state or comprehend—even the infinite calculus of mathematics. The subtle forces of adaptation which have permitted this or that individual to survive in his habitat, his niche, we can but dimly envisage. But what we can see we must utilize to the limit. Only by so doing can we see further.

The application of this ecological principle of all around adaptation, in the medicine of the future, is going to occupy itself more and more with these " hostile impulses " of my opening Haeckel definition, but in a deeper sense than Haeckel ever considered them.

And now in closing let me add that the material which I have sought to bring to your attention, and which I have asked you to consider from a certain point of view, constitutes but a minute fragment in the ecological frame of reference; so minute in my portrayal that I have hesitated even to dignify it by referring it to the field of ecology. Thus I have no statistical data to give it even the verisimilitude of a survey. I have emphasized only a few factors of such an enterprise. For the human aggregate I have but touched upon certain results of faulty adaptation to certain biotic features which are spoken of as psychological or in a less specific sense, sociological.

I have emphasized the essential value of a methodology which in my opinion offers the best approach to an understanding of dynamic drives within the individuals of the human community; drives which because of faulty adaptation result in a host of distorting, mutilating processes within the organs of the individual. Ecology calls these isolates. Medical science gives them a nomenclatural validity and speaks of them as diseases, syndromes, etc.[11]

I have tried to intimate that without such a wide and deep survey many of these major distortions, called organic disease, cannot be comprehended, nor successfully coped with prophylactically or directly.

If I have succeeded, but by allusion, in directing your attention to another mode of approach to the numerous knotty problems which the neo-Hippocratic physician is called upon to disentangle, I shall rest content.

[11] For partial bibliography, see *Am. Jl. Psychiatry*, 92 : 1051, 1936.

INDEX

153

NERVOUS AND MENTAL DISEASE MONOGRAPH SERIES

Founded in 1907 by

SMITH ELY JELLIFFE, M.D., and WILLIAM A. WHITE, M.D.